The Black Death

Other Books in the Turning Points Series:

The Collapse of the Soviet Union
The French Revolution
North American Indian Wars
The Reformation
The Rise of Christianity
The Rise of Nazi Germany
The Spread of Islam

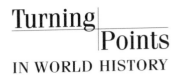

Turning Points
IN WORLD HISTORY

The Black Death

Don Nardo, *Book Editor*

David L. Bender, *Publisher*
Bruno Leone, *Executive Editor*
Bonnie Szumski, *Editorial Director*

Greenhaven Press, Inc., San Diego, California

Every effort has been made to trace the owners of copyrighted material. The articles in this volume may have been edited for content, length, and/or reading level. The titles have been changed to enhance the editorial purpose.

Library of Congress Cataloging-in-Publication Data

The Black Death / Don Nardo, book editor.
    p.   cm. — (Turning points in world history)
    Includes bibliographical references and index.
    ISBN 1-56510-994-5 (pbk. : alk. paper). —
  ISBN 1-56510-995-3 (lib. : alk. paper)
    1. Black Death—Europe—History. 2. Epidemics. I. Nardo, Don, 1947–   . II. Series: Turning points in world history (Greenhaven Press)
RC178.A1B582 1999
614.4'9—dc21
                                                                98-44752
                                                                     CIP

Cover photo: Scala/Art Resource, NY

3/2000 Gen Fund 18.⁰⁰

©1999 by Greenhaven Press, Inc.
P.O. Box 289009, San Diego, CA 92198-9009

Printed in the U.S.A.

Contents

Foreword   9

Introduction: To Stem the Hideous Tide:
The Black Death Decimates Europe   11

Prologue: Disease Epidemics Preceding the Black Death

1. A Natural History of the Plague and Other Early European Diseases *by Robert S. Gottfried*   29
On the eve of the great fourteenth-century disease epidemic known as the Black Death, Europe was expanding in population and increasing its commercial contacts with Asia and Africa. Having no idea what causes disease or how it spreads and living in generally unsanitary conditions, medieval Europeans were wide open to attack by a lethal plague.

Chapter 1: The Black Death Ravages Europe

1. How the Black Death Entered and Spread Through Europe *by Michael W. Dols*   41
Originating in the vast, wild steppes of central Asia, the Black Death spread westward, following the main trade route linking the Far East to the Black Sea region. From there, European traders unwittingly carried the pestilence into the Mediterranean, causing all of Europe to become infected.

2. The Black Death's Grim Death Toll *by Johannes Nohl*   48
The sheer enormity of the disaster wrought by the Black Death is reflected in the huge numbers of people it struck down. According to the fourteenth-century Italian writer Boccaccio, more than half of the inhabitants of the northern Italian city of Florence perished, and mortality figures for other European cities and regions were no less horrific.

3. Medieval Medicine's Response to the Black Death
by Geoffrey Marks   57
When the Black Death struck France, the members of
the Paris College of Physicians, the most prestigious
medical authorities in Europe, declared that the pestilence was caused by noxious, evil vapors produced by
"heavenly disturbances." This was typical of the ignorance of the doctors of the time, who could neither
explain the illness nor save its victims.

4. Anti-Plague Ordinances and Other Social Controls
by Ann G. Carmichael   65
The Black Death did more than kill large numbers of
people. It also altered many social customs, disrupted
trade, and made most people fearful of contact with
strangers. Some towns instituted regulations designed to
limit the spread of the disease, among them travel bans
and crude versions of sanitary laws and quarantines.

5. Atoning for Humanity's Sins: The Flagellants
by Otto Friedrich   73
The flagellants were religious fundamentalists who
marched from town to town, beating themselves with
whips while they sang hymns and said prayers. Their
goal was to convince God to forgive humanity its sins
and thereby end the onslaught of the Black Death. But
when they presented a threat to both religious and secular authorities, their days were numbered.

6. The Black Death Blamed on the Jews
by Barbara W. Tuchman   81
In February 1349, the Christians of Strasbourg, Ger-
many, rounded up the town's 2,000 Jews and burned
them alive. This was only one of hundreds of similar
anti-Semitic acts committed during the great epidemic,
most of them based on a combination of centuries of
ingrained prejudice and the more immediate and completely mistaken belief that the plague had been caused
by Jews poisoning Christian wells.

Chapter 2: The Economic and Cultural Impact of the Black Death

1. **The Black Death's Impact on Economics and Population** *by David Herlihy*   91

In the wake of the huge death toll produced by the Black Death, large tracts of farmland were abandoned or declined in productivity. In ensuing decades and centuries, much of this land came to be used for other purposes, such as pasture for sheep. At the same time, labor losses stimulated the invention of labor-saving devices and other technological advances. These were but two of the many ways the disaster changed the nature of Europe's economy.

2. **Educational, Agricultural, and Architectural Impact of the Black Death** *by Philip Ziegler*   102

Before the Black Death struck Europe, almost all scholarly works were written in Latin, which had long constituted a sort of universal language among the educated. After the disaster, the common tongues of Europe's emerging nations, including English, began to replace Latin. In comparison, a noted scholar argues, the Black Death affected changing architectural styles only slightly.

3. **How the Black Death Affected the Church** *by Frederick F. Cartwright and Michael D. Biddiss*   109

The Christian Church was no more immune to the devastation wrought by the Black Death than other social institutions. Its prestige weakened by the disaster, some within its ranks began calling for reforms, although substantial changes did not occur until the Reformation, some two centuries later.

Epilogue: The Plague and Other Killer Diseases in Modern Times

1. **The New Epidemic** *by Arno Karlen*   115

The world has not seen the last of deadly infectious disease epidemics. Although not on the scale of the

Black Death in the 1300s, AIDS, ebola, exotic influenza, and a host of new and old diseases kill millions of people worldwide each year. And new microbial killers will surely appear in coming years, seemingly out of nowhere, as AIDS and ebola did, presenting ever-new challenges to medical science.

Appendix: Excerpts from Original Documents
  Pertaining to the Black Death   127
Chronology   165
For Further Research   167
Index   170

Foreword

Certain past events stand out as pivotal, as having effects and outcomes that change the course of history. These events are often referred to as turning points. Historian Louis L. Snyder provides this useful definition:

> A turning point in history is an event, happening, or stage which thrusts the course of historical development into a different direction. By definition a turning point is a great event, but it is even more—a great event with the explosive impact of altering the trend of man's life on the planet.

History's turning points have taken many forms. Some were single, brief, and shattering events with immediate and obvious impact. The invasion of Britain by William the Conqueror in 1066, for example, swiftly transformed that land's political and social institutions and paved the way for the rise of the modern English nation. By contrast, other single events were deemed of minor significance when they occurred, only later recognized as turning points. The assassination of a little-known European nobleman, Archduke Franz Ferdinand, on June 28, 1914, in the Bosnian town of Sarajevo was such an event; only after it touched off a chain reaction of political-military crises that escalated into the global conflict known as World War I did the murder's true significance become evident.

Other crucial turning points occurred not in terms of a few hours, days, months, or even years, but instead as evolutionary developments spanning decades or even centuries. One of the most pivotal turning points in human history, for instance—the development of agriculture, which replaced nomadic hunter-gatherer societies with more permanent settlements—occurred over the course of many generations. Still other great turning points were neither events nor developments, but rather revolutionary new inventions and innovations that significantly altered social customs and ideas, military tactics, home life, the spread of knowledge, and the human condition in general. The developments of writing, gunpowder, the printing press, antibiotics, the electric light, atomic energy, television, and the computer, the last two of which have recently ushered in the world-altering information age, represent only some of these innovative turning points.

Each anthology in the Greenhaven Turning Points in World History series presents a group of essays chosen for their accessibility. The anthology's structure also enhances this accessibility. First, an introductory essay provides a general overview of the principal events and figures involved, placing the topic in its historical context. The essays that follow explore various aspects in more detail, some targeting political trends and consequences, others social, literary, cultural, and/or technological ramifications, and still others pivotal leaders and other influential figures. To aid the reader in choosing the material of immediate interest or need, each essay is introduced by a concise summary of the contributing writer's main themes and insights.

In addition, each volume contains extensive research tools, including a collection of excerpts from primary source documents pertaining to the historical events and figures under discussion. In the anthology on the French Revolution, for example, readers can examine the works of Rousseau, Voltaire, and other writers and thinkers whose championing of human rights helped fuel the French people's growing desire for liberty; the French *Declaration of the Rights of Man and Citizen*, presented to King Louis XVI by the French National Assembly on October 2, 1789; and eyewitness accounts of the attack on the royal palace and the horrors of the Reign of Terror. To guide students interested in pursuing further research on the subject, each volume features an extensive bibliography, which for easy access has been divided into separate sections by topic. Finally, a comprehensive index allows readers to scan and locate content efficiently. Each of the anthologies in the Greenhaven Turning Points in World History series provides students with a complete, detailed, and enlightening examination of a crucial historical watershed.

Introduction: To Stem the Hideous Tide: The Black Death Decimates Europe

"Many ended their lives in the public streets," writes the fourteenth-century literary master Giovanni Boccaccio,

> while many others who died in their homes were discovered dead by their neighbors only by the smell of their decomposing bodies. The city was full of corpses. The dead were usually given the same treatment by their neighbors. . . . They would drag the corpse out of the home and place it in front of the doorstep, where, usually in the morning, quantities of dead bodies could be seen by any passerby. . . . The dead were honored with no tears or candles or funeral mourners; in fact, things had reached such a point that the people who died were cared for as we care for goats today.[1]

This passage constitutes only a small part of Boccaccio's long and vivid description of the horrors visited on the Italian city of Florence in 1348 as the disease now referred to as the Black Death ravaged Europe. That continent had endured terrible plagues in the past, but these had mostly been confined to individual cities or regions. None could compare in scale and ferocity to the Black Death, which spread relentlessly from city to city and country to country, consuming and devastating whole societies, killing first thousands, then tens of thousands, then millions. Modern scholars place the overall death toll at a minimum of 25 million, about a third of Europe's total population at the time.

Yet that staggering death toll represented only part of the devastation wrought by the Black Death. The disease seemed to kill indiscriminately. Often it wiped out whole families or entire neighborhoods and villages; yet in many other instances, people who had been in close contact with those infected did not contract the pestilence and unaccountably survived. Because no one knew what it was or, more importantly, how to escape or defend against it, the disease spread fear—fear so overwhelming that it frequently eroded the basic bonds of civilized life. "This disaster," as Boccaccio writes,

> had struck such fear into the hearts of men and women that brother abandoned brother, uncle abandoned nephew, sister left brother, and very often wife abandoned husband, and—even worse, almost unbelievable—fathers and mothers neglected to tend and care for their children as if they were not their own.[2]

In time, these bonds were reestablished. But the way that Europeans viewed death, God, and life in general had been permanently altered. Why had doctors and especially priests, God's servants on the earth, been unable to stem the plague's hideous tide? Was the disease indeed a punishment inflicted by God to punish humanity's sins? Or did God simply not care what happened to human beings? In his widely acclaimed book about the Black Death, noted scholar Philip Ziegler states:

> If one were to seek . . . one generalization . . . to catch the mood of the Europeans in the second half of the fourteenth century, it would be that they were enduring a crisis of faith. Assumptions which had been taken for granted for centuries were now in question, the very framework of men's reasoning seemed to be breaking up. And though the Black Death was far from being the only cause, the anguish and disruption which it had inflicted made the greatest single contribution to the disintegration of an age.[3]

In its wake, then, the Black Death left Europe not only depopulated but also psychologically altered. And economic, social, religious, legal, and educational systems underwent similar transformations, contributing significantly to the already ongoing changeover from medieval to modern civilization. For these reasons, the onset of the Black Death in the fourteenth century marked a crucial turning point in world history.

What Was It?

Most modern historians accept the idea that the medieval Black Death was bubonic plague, primarily a disease of wild rodents. Identified and described by biologists in the 1890s, it has struck humanity several times in the modern era (although never as severely as in the 1300s) and its ecology is now well understood. First, a strain of deadly bacteria, called *Yersinia pestis*,[4] multiplies rapidly in the blood of infected rodents. Fleas infesting the rodents then ingest the bacteria. Several types of flea can carry the disease, but the most common is *Xenopsylla cheopis*, the rat flea, which, as its name suggests, usually remains content to make its home in rat fur. Unfortunately for humans, another scenario occasionally transpires, as scholar Rosemary Horrox explains:

> Under normal conditions the plague makes the transition from rodents to humans relatively rarely, in part because the wild rodents in which the disease is endemic [largely restricted to] are unlikely to come into sufficiently close contact with people for their fleas to move onto a human host. Thus, although plague exists today among the rodent population in parts of the United States, there have been only a handful of cases of people contracting the disease. What seems to have happened in the mid-fourteenth century is that ecological changes in central Asia (where wild rodents formed a reservoir of the disease) drove the infected animals out of their existing habitats and into closer proximity to human settlement, allowing the disease to become endemic among the local rat population and facilitating the movement of fleas to human hosts.[5]

Once on human skin, the fleas bite and then, prior to feeding, regurgitate plague bacteria directly into the tiny open wound. Inside their new host, the bacteria move through the lymphatic system to the lymph nodes and there multiply, forming large colonies. Within three to eight days the resultant swelling creates the egg-shaped lumps, or buboes, usually in the groin or underarms, that characterize the disease. After another three or four days, the bacteria reach the bloodstream and move to the vital organs, especially the spleen and lungs, causing dark spots on and then bleeding from the skin, bleeding from the bowels, and in most cases, if untreated, death.

The reason for the modern consensus that the Black Death was bubonic plague is that many medieval writers described symptoms identical or at least very similar to those of plague. Yet a few scholars remain unconvinced that plague, or at least plague as it is now known, was the culprit. One prominent dissenter, for example, British zoologist Graham Twigg, is puzzled by the fact that no medieval writers mention epizootics, or mass outbreaks, and subsequent deaths, of infected rats.[6] All modern outbreaks of plague in humans have been preceded by conspicuous examples of such dyings. Might this mean that the Black Death was not bubonic plague but rather some other disease with similar symptoms?[7]

In fact, the dissenters point out, other diseases *can* display symptoms like those of plague. It has also been suggested that what appears in retrospect to have been a single disease might actually have been two or more diseases working in tandem. According to the highly respected historian David Herlihy:

> Unfortunately for certain identification, many fevers share these traits [symptoms], but no one of them, including bubonic plague, shows them all. A fulminant [sudden and severe] rash appears in cases of typhoid and typhus fever, and both can sustain epidemics. Other symptoms—the presence of skin lesions over long periods, the spitting of blood, even inflammation of the lymph glands—suggest forms of tuberculosis. Perhaps different diseases were responsible for epidemics of different years [during the mid–fourteenth-century outbreak]. Perhaps too they sometimes worked together . . . to produce the staggering mortalities. Finally, the plague bacilli [bacteria] may have taken on variant forms, aping other diseases in the pathology they produced. . . . The plague bacillus . . . probably has not even today exhausted its capacity to evolve into new forms. It is not at all certain that the diseases we observe today are the same that troubled our ancestors.[8]

Many scholars discount these arguments. Rosemary Horrox, for instance, insists that, to thrive and spread, bubonic plague needs infected fleas more than it does infected rats. "An infected flea can remain alive for at least eighty days away from its rodent host," she points out, "long enough to travel considerable distances in traded goods."[9] She suggests that the Black Death was indeed plague, but that it was a mutant form that was much more virulent than the strains seen in modern times. Nevertheless, these ongoing arguments underscore the little-known fact that the Black Death's identity has yet to be confirmed to everyone's satisfaction.

A Trail of Destruction

Whatever the exact nature of the disease or diseases involved, scholars generally agree about how the epidemic reached Europe and spread throughout the continent. The earliest known appearance of the Black Death in its great mid–fourteenth-century onslaught was in a Christian community just south of Lake Balkhash (in central Asia, about one thousand miles east of the Caspian Sea). Archaeologists have found a cemetery with an unusually high number of graves dating to the years 1338–1339; three of the gravestones actually identify plague as the cause of death. This, along with other evidence, suggests that the disease originated somewhere in the vast steppes of central Asia.

In the 1340s the Black Death moved southward into India and also westward along the ancient trade route that ran from the Far East, through the Mongol (or Tartar) lands in what is now southern Russia, to the Black Sea region. By 1345 huge numbers of Mongols in the Russian steppes were dying of the disease. Then it reached the Crimea, a peninsula on the northern shores of the Black Sea, where in the winter of 1345–1346 a Mongol chieftain laid siege to the Genoese colony of Kaffa. (At the time, the Genoese, hailing from Genoa, an independent republic in northwestern Italy, were aggressive traders whose ships regularly visited ports all along the coasts of the Black and Mediterranean Seas.) During the siege, the Mongols employed a novel and deadly weapon. According to a contemporary Italian account:

They ordered corpses to be placed in catapults and lobbed into the city in the hope that the intolerable stench would kill everyone inside. What seemed like mountains of dead were thrown into the city, and the Christians could not hide or flee or escape from them, although they dumped as many of the bodies as they could into the sea. . . . One infected man could carry the poison to others, and infect people and places with the disease by look alone. No one knew, or could discover, a means of defence.[10]

After many months of misery, some of the Genoese managed to escape in their ships and sailed toward the Mediterranean. They had no idea that they carried with them a microscopic cargo of death. By 1347 the Black Death had begun to ravage Constantinople, the great Byzantine trading city lying astride the straits connecting the Black and Mediterranean Seas. Because thousands of ships from all over the Mediterranean routinely docked there, it was virtually inevitable that the disease would spread via shipping to the ports of Syria, Palestine, Egypt, northern Africa, Greece, Italy, France, and Spain. And indeed, all of these areas were infected by early 1348. One Byzantine writer claimed, "A plague attacked almost all the seacoasts of the world and killed most of the people."[11] The horror was that this was only a slight exaggeration. In some cities and regions as much as half or more of the population died; only a few cities escaped with a death rate lower than 30 percent.

From Europe's ports, the Black Death next raged inland, moving northward and eastward. Describing its terrifying passage through the French countryside, the contemporary French chronicler Jean de Venette records:

Such an enormous number of people died in 1348 and 1349 that nothing like it has been heard or seen or read about. . . . A healthy person who visited the sick hardly ever escaped death. . . . To be brief, in many places not two men remained alive out of twenty. The mortality was so great that, for a considerable period, more than 500 bodies a day were being taken in carts from the Hotel-Dieu in Paris for burial in the cemetery of the Holy Innocents.[12]

After the disease had decimated northern France, its trail of destruction reached the English Channel, which, contrary to the hopeful expectations of the English, provided no barrier to the contagion. The epidemic struck southern Britain with a fury late in 1348, and by the end of 1349 it had reached the Scottish highlands and eastern Ireland.

At the same time, traders and travelers unwittingly carried the Black Death through what is now Germany and Russia. In 1352 it reached Moscow, where it claimed the lives of the local grand duke and the patriarch of the Russian church, along with untold numbers of less prominent people; then it spread southward and decimated the city of Kiev. Ironically, the lethal contagion had taken a long, circuitous route to Kiev—southward from the Crimea, through the seas to southern Europe, and then northeastward into Russia. As David Herlihy puts it, "Launched at Kaffa in the Crimea, and now attaining Kiev, some 700 kilometers [about 435 miles] to the north, the plague almost closed a deadly noose around Europe."[13]

Many Theories, Few Facts

These frightening events occurred some five hundred years before the discovery of the connection between germs and disease. So, quite understandably, no one in plague-ravaged Europe had any idea what was infecting and killing so many people. Theories abounded, however. The most common explanation for the crisis was that it was a manifestation of God's wrath. "Terrible is God toward the sons of men," wrote an English cleric in September 1348 as the Black Death descended on his land,

> and by his command all things are subdued to the rule of his will. Those whom he loves he censures and chastises; that is, he punishes their shameful deeds in various ways during this mortal life so that they might not be condemned eternally. He often allows plagues, miserable famines, conflicts, wars and other forms of suffering to arise, and uses them to terrify and torment men and so drive out their sins. And thus, indeed, the realm of England, because of the growing pride

and corruption of its subjects, and their numberless sins . . .
is to be oppressed by the pestilences and wretched mortalities of men which have flared up in other regions.[14]

Another Englishman agreed, lamenting, "See how England
mourns, drenched in tears. The people stained by sin, quake
with grief. Plague is killing men and beasts. Why? Because
vices rule unchallenged here."[15] In Italy, Boccaccio echoed
the same refrain, calling the disaster "God's just wrath as a
punishment to mortals for our wicked deeds."[16]

There were other explanations as well, many of them of a
physical nature, although it was often assumed that divine
anger had set them in motion. "Corrupted," "tainted," or
"unclean" air was frequently cited, for instance. In October
1348, a group of French doctors issued a statement in which
they asserted:

> Although major pestilential illnesses can be caused by the
> corruption of water or food . . . yet we still regard illnesses
> proceeding from the corruption of the air as much more
> dangerous. This is because bad air is more noxious than food
> or drink in that it can penetrate quickly to the heart and
> lungs to do its damage. We believe that the present epidemic
> or plague has arisen from air corrupt in its substance, and not
> changed in its attributes. By which we wish it [to] be under-
> stood that air, being pure and clear by nature, can only be-
> come putrid or corrupt by being mixed with something else,
> that is to say, with evil vapours.[17]

This passage underscores the sad fact that medieval doctors had no idea what caused the Black Death and were
equally ignorant of effective methods of treatment. To their
credit, it did become clear to many people, doctors and laymen alike, that the disease was somehow contagious. And
some towns and regions tried restricting travel, imposing
sanitation codes, and implementing quarantines. In May
1348, for example, the Italian town of Pistoia passed several
antiplague ordinances, among them:

> No citizen or resident of Pistoia . . . shall dare or presume to
> go to Pisa or Lucca; and no one shall come to Pistoia from

those places. . . . No one . . . shall dare or presume to bring or fetch to Pistoia . . . any old linen or woollen cloths . . . and the cloth [already here is] to be burned in the public piazza [town square]. . . . The bodies of the dead shall not be removed from the place of death until they have been enclosed in a wooden box, and the lid of planks nailed down so that no stench can escape. . . . To avoid the foul stench which comes from dead bodies each grave shall be dug two and a half arms-length deep. . . . No one, of whatever condition, status or standing, shall dare or presume to bring a corpse into the city, whether coffined [i.e., in a coffin] or not.[18]

In March 1348 authorities in Venice resorted to similar desperate measures. They designated special barges to carry infected persons to isolated islands, buried the dead at least five feet deep in the earth, and imposed a forty-day-long ban on incoming ships, threatening violators with immediate death. These efforts proved futile, however. The Black Death still killed some 60 percent of Venice's inhabitants in the ensuing eighteen months. Similar ordinances and quarantines across Europe were also largely ineffective, mainly because, out of ignorance of the actual transmission mode, they failed to separate infected insects and rodents along with the infected people.

The Jews and the Flagellants

Another common theory, one born out of both extreme fear and ingrained prejudice, was that the epidemic was caused by Jews poisoning wells and other water supplies in an effort to wipe out Christians.[19] "Some wretched men were found in possession of certain powders," reported an Italian commentator in April 1348, "and (whether justly or unjustly, God knows) were accused of poisoning the wells—with the result that anxious men now refuse to drink water from wells. Many were burnt for this and are being burnt daily, for it was ordered that they be punished thus."[20] A German churchman left this horrific account of anti-Semitic persecutions:

The persecution of the Jews began in November 1348, and the first outbreak in Germany was at Sölden, where all the

Jews were burnt on the strength of a rumour that they had poisoned wells and rivers, as was afterwards confirmed by their own confessions. . . . All the Jews between Cologne and Austria were burnt and killed for this crime, young men and maidens and the old along with the rest. And blessed be God who confounded the ungodly who were plotting the extinction of his church. . . . On 20 December in Horw they [the Jews] were burnt in a pit. And when the wood and straw had been consumed, some Jews, both young and old, still remained half alive. The stronger of [the Christians] snatched up cudgels [clubs] and stones and dashed out the brains of those trying to creep out of the fire, and thus compelled those who wanted to escape the fire to descend to hell.[21]

While many people attempted to combat the Black Death by imposing quarantines and sanitation ordinances, restricting travel, and continuing to hound and murder innocent Jews, all to no avail, others appealed directly to God. When earnest prayers seemed to fall on deaf ears, some of the devout joined groups of flagellants (from the word *flagellate*, meaning "to punish by whipping"). Organized battalions of at least two hundred and sometimes as many as a few thousand flagellants marched somberly from town to town. As they entered a town square, they stripped themselves to the waist and beat themselves with whips, often tipped with metal spikes, until they bled. This was intended as a reenactment of the scourging of Christ before his crucifixion; they hoped that this dramatic and painful act of atonement would persuade God to forgive humanity's sins and thus end the continent-wide epidemic. As they thrashed themselves, they cried out, "Spare us, Jesus!," "Forgive us, blessed Mary!"

Meanwhile, the local townspeople who beheld this bizarre spectacle swayed and moaned and wept in sympathy. Or at least at first they did. In time, many became suspicious and fearful of approaching flagellants, who increasingly assumed the role of mediator between God and humanity, and thereby threatened the authority of the priesthood and the Church. Noted scholar Barbara Tuchman explains:

Growing in arrogance, they became overt in antagonism to the

Church. The Masters [leading flagellants] assumed the right to hear confession and grant absolution or impose penance, which not only denied the priests their fee for these services, but challenged ecclesiastical authority at its core. Priests who intervened against them were stoned and the populace was incited to join in the stoning. Opponents were denounced as scorpions and Anti-Christs. . . . The flagellants took possession of churches, disrupted services . . . looted altars, and claimed the power to cast out evil spirits and raise the dead. The movement that began as an attempt through self-inflicted pain to save the world from destruction, caught the infection of power hunger and aimed at taking over the Church.[22]

In response to this growing threat, religious and secular leaders soon joined in a concerted effort to discredit and disband the flagellants. In October 1349 Pope Clement VI called for the arrest of the self-torturers; the prestigious University of Paris declared that they were not, as they claimed, inspired by God; and many local rulers hunted down, arrested, and summarily executed them. Although, thanks to these tactics, most of the flagellant bands had dispersed by 1351, a few survived until as late as 1357.

Economic and Social Alterations

By sheer coincidence, the waning of the flagellant movement roughly coincided with the waning of this greatest of all outbreaks of the Black Death. By early 1351 the disease had largely run its course in most of Europe. Later that year agents for Pope Clement, who desired an overall appraisal of the disaster, calculated the total death toll in Europe at 23,840,000. The accuracy of this figure is uncertain, but based on studies of literary, archaeological, and other evidence, modern scholars contend that it was certainly not any lower and very probably somewhat higher. Making matters worse, more people died in subsequent outbreaks (in 1361, 1369, 1375, and 1390 in England, and on twenty-two occasions between 1348 and 1596 in France); although none of these were nearly as destructive as the 1348 visitation.

It would, of course, be impossible for a catastrophe of this

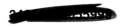

magnitude not to have had powerful and far-reaching effects on the lives of the survivors. And indeed, the social, economic, intellectual, technological, and religious impacts of the Black Death were profound. First, economic and social institutions underwent dramatic alterations. The medieval manorial system, in which wealthy lords living in castles exploited poor peasants who had been tied to their lands for generations, had already begun to weaken before the epidemic's onslaught. That onslaught finally brought the old order crashing down. Massive depopulation left rich landowners with far fewer workers than they needed to keep up their domains and turn a profit; those workers now demanded and won the right to rent or lease the lands on which they had formerly been little more than slaves. Rutgers University historian Robert Gottfried elaborates:

> The Black Death brought a crisis to the nobility.... Depopulation meant widespread mobility and fluidity for those not tied to the land. The value of agricultural products began to fall, and it stayed low relative to that of industrial goods until the sixteenth century; at the same time, depopulation made agricultural workers scarce and, thus, much more valuable. Wages rose rapidly.... At Cuxham Manor in England, a plowman who was paid 2 shillings a week in 1347 received 7 shillings in 1349, and 10 shillings ... by 1350. The result was a dramatic rise in standards of living for those in the lower [social classes].... Day laborers not only received higher wages, but asked for and got lunches of meat pies and golden ale.[23]

As John Gower, an English country gentleman, complained in 1375:

> The world goeth fast from bad to worse, when shepherd and cowherd ... demand more for their labor than the master-baliff was wont to take in days gone by. Labor is now at so high a price that he who will order his business aright must pay five or six shillings now for what cost him two in former times. ... Ha! ... The poor and small folk ... demand to be better fed than their masters.[24]

In a desperate effort to maintain the traditional economic

and social order, the landed classes passed laws and imposed new taxes designed to keep the lower classes "in their place." But this only led to peasant uprisings, one of the biggest of which occurred in England in 1381. Upwards of one hundred thousand peasants marched on London and demanded to see King Richard II. According to English chronicler Henry Knighton:

> They directed their way to the Tower [of London] where the king was surrounded by a great throng of knights, esquires, and others [attempting to protect him]. . . . They [the peasants] complained that they had been seriously oppressed by many hardships and that their condition of servitude was unbearable, and that they neither could nor would endure it longer. The king, for the sake of peace, and on account of the violence of the times, yielding to their petition, granted them a charter . . . to the effect that all men in the kingdom . . . should be free and of free condition.[25]

Later that year, the king and his nobles nullified this charter. Yet the English underclass had made substantial gains. The crown was forced to reduce taxes and thereafter refrained from passing laws designed to keep workers' wages low. By 1400 the old manorial system had all but disappeared in England.

Technological and Religious Changes

As Europe's economic order rapidly changed, the value of land decreased. Capital investments, such as the purchase of oxen, seed, and fertilizers to make land more productive (or better tools and machines to enable artisans to work more efficiently) were also cheaper. These developments, combined with the increased cost of labor, stimulated the invention of new labor-saving devices. Late medieval times therefore witnessed sudden and impressive advances in technology. Herlihy cites the example of the invention of printing with movable type:

> The growth of universities in the twelfth and thirteenth centuries and the expanding numbers of literate laymen generated a strong demand for books. Numerous scribes were employed

to copy manuscripts. . . . As long as wages were low, this method of reproduction based on intensive human labor was satisfactory enough. But the late medieval population plunge raised labor costs and also raised the premium to be claimed by the one who could devise a cheaper way of reproducing books. Johann Gutenberg's invention of printing on the basis of movable metal type in 1453 was only the culmination of many experiments carried on across the previous century.[26]

Another example of a technological advance stimulated by the changing economy was a virtual revolution in maritime transport. Investors sank large amounts of capital into building bigger ships with much improved construction techniques and new advances in navigation. These vessels required smaller crews (making them less expensive to operate), carried more cargo, and could remain at sea longer, greatly increasing the profit potential.

Like technology, medicine, which had been powerless to deal with the Black Death, made impressive advances in the years following its great European assault. Faced with a clear and vital need to understand and overcome their past failure, European doctors began hands-on studies of the human body, a practice unknown since the days of the renowned ancient Greek physician Galen. Dissecting human cadavers, which had long been banned, became increasingly widespread, and by the end of the fourteenth century notable strides had been made in the science of anatomy. In addition, surgery, long excluded from the medical curriculum at European universities, became a staple of advanced medical study. A thorough understanding of the causes of disease was still many centuries away; but the new medical establishment created in the post–Black Death century began to lay the groundwork for the development of the scientific method that would eventually lead to that understanding.

Still another way the Black Death impacted European society was to change the way people viewed the Church, the clergy, and their own relationship with God. Large numbers of Europeans believed that priests and bishops (many of whom had died in the epidemic) had been unable to intercede with God and stop the plague; the Church therefore suffered a measurable loss of prestige. After the epidemic, most Christians remained devout and still supported the Church, to be sure. But many came to believe that they could have an individual relationship with God without the need for a priest as an intermediary. Thousands who before would have asked a priest to pray for them now prayed for themselves, for example. There was also a substantial upsurge in individual good works, such as charitable contributions to hospitals, monasteries, and the poor. And huge numbers sought salvation by going on long and often dangerous pilgrimages to shrines in Rome, Jerusalem, and other holy sites.

A Civilization Scared out of Its Wits

Perhaps this veritable avalanche of charitable and godly actions was in a way a sort of overcompensation, a large-scale attempt to appease God and thereby ensure that He would never again vent His wrath so terribly on humanity. Perhaps it was also a way for millions of people to prove to themselves that they still believed in God. For it is likely that during the crisis itself some, if not many, momentarily doubted the existence of a god who could strike down the innocent along with the guilty, priests and nuns along with murderers. Afterward, based on the assumption that the epidemic had been a divine punishment, it was simply not worth the risk of doubting God's existence. "The generation that survived the plague could not believe but did not dare deny," quips Philip Ziegler. "It groped myopically [having little or no notion of what lay ahead] towards the future, with one nervous eye always peering over its shoulder towards the past."[27]

Thus, medieval civilization was in a very real sense scared, almost out of its wits, into new modes of thinking and acting. Combined with other social, economic, and technological factors that followed, these changes soon ushered in a new civilization in Europe, the one we call "modern." Like the fall of Rome, the invention of gunpowder, and the American Revolution, the onset of the Black Death in the fourteenth century was a major historical watershed because, put simply, in its wake nothing was ever quite the same again.

Notes

1. Giovanni Boccaccio, *The Decameron*, trans. Mark Musa and Peter Bondanella, New York: W.W. Norton, 1982, pp. 10–11.

2. Boccaccio, *The Decameron*, p. 9.

3. Philip Ziegler, *The Black Death*. New York: Harper and Row, 1969, p. 279.

4. The germ is named for Alexandre Yersin, the Swiss microbiologist who isolated it in 1894 and went on to develop a serum for treating the disease.

5. Rosemary Horrox, ed., *The Black Death*. Manchester, England: Manchester University Press, 1994, p. 5.

6. See Graham Twigg, *The Black Death: A Biological Reappraisal*. New York: Schocken Books, 1984, pp. 19–24, 90–112.

7. Twigg first proposed anthrax, a disease that today usually affects only cattle but that on occasion infects humans. Later he modified his position, suggesting an unknown disease characterized by "an air-borne organism of high infectivity and virulence, having a short incubation period and being spread by respiratory means."

8. David Herlihy, *The Black Death and the Transformation of the West*, ed. Samuel K. Cohn Jr. Cambridge, MA: Harvard University Press, 1997, pp. 30–31.

9. Horrox, *The Black Death*, p. 7.

10. Gabriele de Mussis, *Historia de Morbo*, quoted in Horrox, *The Black Death*, p. 17.

11. Nicephorus Gregoras, *Ecclesiastical History*, quoted in Herlihy, *The Black Death*, p. 24.

12. Jean de Venette, *Chronicle*, trans. Rosemary Horrox, in Horrox, *The Black Death*, pp. 55–56.

13. Herlihy, *The Black Death*, p. 25.

14. Prior of Christchurch, *Terribilis*, quoted in Horrox, *The Black Death*, pp. 113–14.

15. Quoted in Horrox, *The Black Death*, p. 126.

16. Boccaccio, *The Decameron*, p. 6.

17. *Report of the Paris Medical Faculty, October 1348*, quoted in Horrox, *The Black Death*, pp. 160–61.

18. *Anti-Plague Ordinances of Pistoia, 1348*, quoted in Horrox, *The Black Death*, pp. 195–96.

19. Charges of well-poisoning were nothing new. When a plague struck Athens, Greece, in circa 430 B.C., many Athenians accused their enemies, the Spartans, of poisoning their wells. Later, in the midst of an epidemic (of unknown identity) in France in 1320–1321, it was widely believed that lepers, Muslims, and Jews were conspiring together to poison water supplies and thereby cripple Christian towns. Thus, when the Black Death struck Europe in the late 1340s, the Jews became a familiar and easy scapegoat.

20. Louis Heyligen, "Letter of April 27, 1348," quoted in Horrox, *The Black Death*, p. 45.

21. Heinrich Truchess von Diessenhoven, *Persecution of the Jews*, quoted in Horrox, *The Black Death*, pp. 208–209.

22. Barbara Tuchman, *A Distant Mirror: The Calamitous 14th Century.* New York: Knopf, 1978, p. 115.

23. Robert Gottfried, *The Black Death: Natural and Human Disaster in Medieval Europe.* New York: Macmillan, 1983, p. 94.

24. *Vox Clamantis,* quoted in Otto Freidrich, *The End of the World: A History.* New York: Fromm International, 1986, p. 135.

25. Henry Knighton, *History of England,* quoted in Leon Bernard and Theodore B. Hodges, eds., *Readings in European History.* New York: Macmillan, 1958, pp. 214–15.

26. Herlihy, *The Black Death,* pp. 49–50.

27. Ziegler, *The Black Death,* p. 279.

Disease Epidemics Preceding the Black Death

Turning Points

IN WORLD HISTORY

A Natural History of the Plague and Other Early European Diseases

Robert S. Gottfried

This informative essay is by Rutgers University history professor Robert Gottfried, whose book, The Black Death: Natural and Human Disaster in Medieval Europe, is one of the most widely read on the subject. He begins by describing the state of Europe on the eve of the fourteenth-century onslaught of the Black Death, then explains how social, sanitary, and other conditions in the ancient and medieval world greatly facilitated the spread of disease. Next, Gottfried examines the nature, spread, and death tolls of the most common infectious diseases of these times—smallpox, measles, leprosy, tuberculosis, and bubonic plague. His discussion of the latter, especially in relation to the fourteenth century, is based on the widely, although not completely, accepted assumption that the Black Death was indeed bubonic plague. Note that Gottfried frequently uses two technical terms routinely associated with disease epidemics. "Virulent" means extremely contagious and deadly; an "epizoötic" is a lethal epidemic affecting a large animal population.

Like all infectious diseases, the Black Death has a natural history and can be properly understood only in that context. First, there is environment. Anyone traveling through Europe today would find it hard to imagine what the continent looked like a thousand years ago. There were no sprawling urban and industrial complexes, the outstanding characteristic of the last century, and surprisingly few towns of any size.

Towns were usually far apart, located next to the sea or astride great rivers. By the middle of the twelfth century, a few urban centers in Italy and the Netherlands, and perhaps Paris, had fifty thousand or more people, but most claimed a thousand or so inhabitants. Nine out of ten Europeans lived in still smaller settlements, nucleated villages of hamlets of a few hundred people, fifteen to twenty miles apart. Both town and village were small and cramped, with woefully inadequate sanitation and transportation facilities. Ironically, in the confines of their small but isolated settlements, most people lived close together and had little privacy.

Surrounding the villages were the fields, pastures, and woodlands from which most people squeezed their subsistence. By 1250 or so, field and pasture had come to dominate Europe's landscape, but, until at least the mid-twelfth century, the extent and density of the woodlands characterized the European environment. . . .

Causes and Transmission of Disease

A second consideration in studying disease is causation. All epidemics, plague included, are caused by parasites that have relations with other, usually larger organisms. This process is a natural part of human and animal ecology. A third factor, and one of paramount concern to man, is toxicity. Epidemiologists generally distinguish between lethal and nonlethal diseases. Nonlethal infections are usually "old" and well-established. Often, they are only mildly deleterious to their hosts, thus ensuring a steady supply of victims. By contrast, those spectacular diseases that, periodically burst onto the historical stage, killing large numbers of people, are caused by newer parasites that have yet to establish an equilibrium with their hosts. An example of an older disease is malaria; the plasmodium [microscopic parasite] that causes it is debilitating, but generally not fatal. An example of a newer disease is pneumonic plague, which is 95% to 100% fatal. Both diseases have been significant in the past, but because of the plague's enormous mortality, it has had far greater impact.

A fourth concern regarding infectious diseases—and, indeed, an important way of distinguishing one from another—is their means of transmission. One such mechanism is direct contact between people, usually via the respiratory system. Diseases so disseminated include influenza, diphtheria, measles, and pneumonic plague. Respiratory diseases are highly communicable, virtually impossible to prevent, and closely related to human population density. Consequently, they were common in the cities and towns of medieval Europe. A second mechanism of dissemination comprises enteric diseases, those spread through the digestive system; among them are dysentery, diarrhea, typhoid, and cholera. Like respiratory afflictions, enteric ailments were very common throughout the Middle Ages. They often reflected social conditions, especially poor sanitation. Because of this, and in contrast to respiratory diseases, enteric diseases can be eliminated rather easily through basic improvements in public health.

Diseases Passed from Animals to Humans

Diseases are spread in at least two other fashions. One is through venereal contact, the prime example being the treponema infections, especially syphilis, and gonorrhea. The causative organisms of venereal ailments are highly vulnerable when exposed, even in temperate environments, and were less frequent in the Middle Ages than were either respiratory or enteric diseases. A fourth group, however, was very common—diseases transferred to humans from animal hosts, with animals acting either as intermediaries, as with malaria or typhus, or as primary or secondary epizoötic victims, as with bubonic plague. The role of animals in the spread of diseases can be crucial: humans share 65 different diseases with dogs; 50 with cattle; 46 with sheep and goats; 42 with pigs; 35 with horses; 32 with rats and mice; and 26 with poultry. While not as common as respiratory or enteric diseases, those transmitted by animals are usually more lethal, since most viruses and bacteria, the organisms that actually cause infection, gain in virulence as they pass through the chain of hosts.

In addition to their virulence, diseases facilitated by animal intermediaries are important for other reasons. They represent still another disease classification and interpretation in that their dissemination and frequency are based primarily on the animal hosts rather than on humans. Bubonic plague provides a good example. When a rodent population in which plague is enzoötic, that is, indigenous, begins to multiply and reaches a certain population density, there is a concentrated transfer among the rodents of parasites—fleas, in this case—and bacteria. The result is usually an epizoötic among the rodents, which sometimes leads to an epidemic of bubonic plague. Some scholars have suggested that communicable diseases are a basic part of the human environment and a function of the population density, and that civilization and disease travel hand in hand. Accordingly, the incidence of a given epidemic would hinge on patterns of human settlement. This is indeed the case with respiratory, enteric, and venereal diseases, but it is not so with those diseases spread by animal intermediaries. The latter are primarily dependent on factors exogenous to civilization, such as climate and rodent and insect population density and ecology. There is great danger when studying the history of infectious diseases in . . . overemphasizing the human element. In many epidemic diseases, humans are most effective as carriers when entering new ecospheres, such as the Americas in the sixteenth century, where they brought smallpox and measles, rather than in areas of older inhabitation, such as Europe in the Middle Ages.

Immunity

Another key characteristic in the development of infectious diseases is immunity. Humans have complex mechanisms for defending themselves against pathogens, the microorganisms that cause disease. Individual resistance varies with many factors, such as number of protective antibodies—the proteins generated in reaction to the disease toxins introduced into the bloodstream. Immunity is either innate or acquired; if acquired, it is either active or passive. Active immunity comes when the host generates his own defenses, passive when generated defenses are introduced. Passive immunity is often only temporary. In the Middle Ages, active immunity was particularly important in determining the extent and intensity of an epidemic. Some infections, especially respiratory types such as smallpox and measles, do not change a great deal in their etiology. Hence, survival from an initial attack confers a degree of immunity, limiting recurrence to those members of society born after the last epidemic. Diseases for which there was immunity had less of an impact on medieval Europe than did more complex, multiple infections such as dysentery, influenza, and plague, for which immunity is quite limited, if it exists at all.

The Ancient Disease Pool

Medieval infectious diseases were an inheritance from the classical world. Between about 500 B.C. and A.D. 550 there were extensive contacts between the animal populations and the civilizations of China, Central Asia, India, the Upper Nile, and the Mediterranean Basin. As a result . . . there was a general confluence of Eurasian and African disease pools which, by the sixth century A.D., brought to the Mediterranean Basin most of the important diseases that can survive in temperate climates. To be sure, this proliferation of diseases took a long time. With a few exceptions, such as the Athenian Plague of the fifth century B.C., the classical world was remarkably free from major, deadly epidemics. This was fundamental to its steady population growth, which continued almost unabated until the second century A.D. But this biological peace was deceptive; in fact, the peripatetic [interconnected] character of ancient empires acted as a conduit and incubator for future disease patterns. An example was the . . . commerce and communications established by the Romans late in the first century B.C. This included their famed road system and, even more important, network of commercial sea routes. The sea routes converged on the Levantine [Palestinian] Coast, then branched east across the northern Arabian Peninsula to the Arabian Sea, the Indian Ocean, and South Asia; and west to Italy, southern Gaul, and Iberia [Spain], whence goods proceeded inland via major river valleys such as the Rhone. Sea travel was relatively quick and, with good weather, all Mediterranean ports were just a few days apart. Thus, a person who seemed well on embarkation could fall sick en route, infect fellow passengers, and then spread the disease hundreds of miles from its point of origin. Further, cargoes were often bulky enough to conceal potential insect and rodent intermediaries. This, coupled with the linking of south and central Asia, the Middle East, the Nile Delta, and the European coast along the Mediterranean, brought about the fruition of disease pools.

From the second through the sixth centuries A.D., three new and lethal infections emerged from this disease pool, bringing an end to the ecological stability of the ancient world. The first began in 165 and persisted until 180, striking Italy and the western part of the Roman Empire. It seems to have been brought west by Roman legionnaires and probably marks the introduction into Mediterranean Europe of smallpox. . . . Smallpox is one of man's most communicable diseases and can be very deadly to a population with no innate immunity. This was the case in the Roman Empire. The [second-century Greek] physician Galen estimated that between a quarter and a third of Italy's population died during the 15 years after it appeared. But because the smallpox virus changes little and survival of an attack generally confers immunity, its role in the Middle Ages was limited to areas it had yet to visit and to those who never had had it—primarily children. Thus, it was as a killer of children that smallpox made its biggest mark in the medieval world.

Smallpox was joined in 251 by the second of the great epidemic diseases, marking the classical/medieval disease watershed. This disease was the "Antonine Plague," probably measles. . . .

At its height, measles allegedly killed 5000 people a day in Rome, and it remained a major menace until about 260. Measles is like smallpox in many ways and the two diseases were not distinguished by European doctors until the sixteenth century. It is caused by a virus, transmitted via the respiratory system, and highly lethal to a population with little or no immunity. As is the case with smallpox, however, survival of a measles attack confers immunity from future visitations. Thus, it, too, was primarily a childhood affliction in the Middle Ages. Nevertheless, it is important not to diminish the effects of either disease, especially in their initial appearances. Measles depleted the population, hastened the desertion of many rural areas (particularly in the grain-producing regions of Sicily and North Africa), and cut the rolls of the Roman army and taxpayers. It caused at least a temporary reduction in East-West trade and, with smallpox, has formed the cornerstone of a major theory of the decline of the Roman Empire.

How Plague Spreads to Humans

Important as smallpox and measles were in the natural history of infectious disease, their combined role was dwarfed by the arrival in 541 of a third disease. This was plague, caused by a complex series of bacterial strains called *Yersinia pestis*. Plague's etiology helps to explain its historical importance; *Y. pestis's* toxicity varies, but the disease is always highly lethal. Under normal circumstances, it lives in the digestive tract of fleas, particularly the rat fleas *Xenopsylla cheopis* and *Cortophylus fasciatus*, but it can also live in the human flea, *Pulex irritans*. Periodically and for reasons that epidemiologists still do not fully understand, the bacilli multiply in the flea's stomach in numbers large enough to cause a blockage, thus threatening the flea with starvation. The "blocked flea," while feeding, regurgitates into its victims large numbers of *Y. pestis* bacilli. This process is crucial to plague's progress; furthermore, *Y. pestis* cannot pass through healthy skin, but only through a break in the surface.

Dozens of rodents carry plague. Among them are tarbagons, marmots, and susliks in Asia, prairie dogs and ground squirrels in America, and gerbels and mice in Africa. Generally living in networks of tunnels just beneath the earth's surface, these rodents can be very numerous. In the Volga steppe in south Russia, an average of 325,000 susliks per four square miles has been estimated. In Europe, rats, especially the black rat, *Rattus rattus*, have been most important carriers. Black rats are quite sedentary and rarely move more than 200 meters from their nests. Because they live so close to humans, they are most dangerous to them. An excellent climber, *R. rattus* was well-suited to both the thatched roofs of peasant dwellings and the high roof beams and dark corners of urban houses. But, important as black rats were in the dissemination of plague, it is essential to emphasize that they were not the only secondary carriers. Along with the other rodents already mentioned, additional secondary vector hosts included virtually all household and barnyard animals save the horse, whose odor apparently repels even starving blocked fleas.

When *Y. pestis* is enzoötic, that is, endemic to a rodent population, it is called silvatic plague. Silvatic plague is crucial to human epidemics because its presence in a rodent population provides a reservoir, or focus, in which the disease can survive for extended periods of time. Reservoirs may help explain the cyclic occurrence of plague, which ultimately made it so important in the Middle Ages. *Y. pestis* is able to live in the dark, moist environment of rodent burrows even after the rodents have been killed by an epizoötic, or epidemic. Thus, if a new rodent community replaces the old one, the plague chain can be revived.

The fleas carrying *Y. pestis* turn to humans only after their supply of secondary hosts has diminished. Most secondary hosts can tolerate a modest proportion of *Y. pestis* in their bloodstreams, but when the bacilli multiply and invade the pulmonary or nervous systems, the secondary hosts succumb. The fleas then seek a new host—and sometimes that host is a human being. Humans, then, are not a preferred host for *Y. pestis*, but rather, the victims of an animal epizoötic. In effect, humans are victims of changes in insect and rodent ecology.

The Three Kinds of Plague

There are three principal varieties of plague—bubonic, pneumonic, and septicaemic. Bubonic is by far the most common and therefore the most important of the three. Its incubation period from the time of infection to the appearance of the first symptoms is generally about six days. The initial symptom, a blackish, often gangrenous pustule at the point of the bite, is followed by an enlargement of the lymph nodes in the armpits, groin, or neck, depending on the place of the flea bite. Next, subcutaneous [below the skin] hemorrhaging occurs, causing the purplish blotches called buboes, from which bubonic plague takes it name. The hemorrhaging produces cell necrosis and intoxication of the nervous system, ultimately leading to neurological and psychological disorders, which may explain the *danse* macabre rituals that accompanied the Black Death. Bubonic plague is the least toxic of all plague types, but it is still highly lethal, killing 50% to 60% of its victims.

Pneumonic plague is unique in that it can be transmitted directly from person to person. This is in part the result of pneumonic plague's peculiar etiology, for it seems to occur only when there is a sharp temperature drop and the infection moves into the lungs. After the two-to-three-day incubation period, there is a rapid fall in body temperature, followed by a severe cough and consolidation in the lungs, rapid cyanosis [dark discoloration of the skin], and the discharge of bloody sputum [saliva and mucus]. The sputum contains *Y. pestis*, making transmission airborne and thus direct from human to human. Neurological difficulties and coma follow infection, with death coming in 95% to 100% of the cases. Therefore, while pneumonic plague is less frequent than bubonic, it is far more virulent.

Like bubonic plague, septicaemic plague is insect-borne, but its precise etiology and occasional appearance in selected epidemics have not been adequately explained. It is known that in septicaemic plague *Y. pestis* bacilli enter the bloodstream of victims in massive numbers. A rash forms within hours and death occurs within a day, before the buboes even have time to form. This type of plague is always fatal, but it is very rare and, because it is present in the bloodstream in such large quantities, it can be transmitted by the human flea, *P. irritans*, and even by the human body louse.

There are peculiar environmental conditions that determine the presence and virulence of plague epidemics. First, there are factors of insect and rodent ecology. The appropriate fleas and rodents must live near people. . . . Climate also plays an important role. The rat flea *X. cheopis* is quite hardy; it can survive for between six months and a year without a rodent host in dung, an abandoned rat's nest, or even textile bales. But it is active only at temperatures of 15°C–20°C, with 90%–95% humidity. Cold limits the flea's activity, while heat retards its productivity, and humidity of less than 70% kills it. These climatic factors limit most plague outbreaks to particular seasons in different parts of the Western world. In western Europe, for example, it generally comes in late summer and early autumn. It is important to stress that an outbreak of plague occurs only in confluence with a variety of environmental conditions.

Plague may be the most virulent of the human infectious diseases. But, historically, its frequency is even more important than its virulence. Plague comes not in isolated epidemics, but rather, in pandemics. A pandemic is a linked series of epidemics that strike in cyclic fashion. It occurs when *Y. pestis* has been established in the local rodent population, as discussed above, and is itself determined by climatic and ecological conditions. Once a pandemic is present, plague epidemics will recur in intervals of between 2 and 20 years. Hence, epidemics will strike at least once in every generation and act as a regular population check. Plague is unique among epidemic diseases in its deadly combination of virulence and frequency. . . .

Europe on the Eve of the Black Death

From the late eighth through the mid-fourteenth century, Europe was remarkably free from most epidemic diseases. . . .

[But] Europe's relatively disease-free era ended abruptly in the mid-fourteenth century. Population had increased about 300% from the tenth to the mid-thirteenth century to 75–80 million, higher than it had been for close to a thousand years. Militant imperialism had extended the boundaries of the Christian West into Russia, Iberia, and Palestine. Internal European trade and travel had improved considerably with the opening of new Alpine passes, the establishment of a direct sea-link between the Italian and Netherlandish cities, and the integration of the Baltic and North Sea hinterlands with the rest of the continent. Most important in epidemiological terms, closer connections were being forged between Europe, Asia, and Africa. To ease a bullion shortage, Italian merchants turned to Arab middlemen for access to sub-Saharan gold supplies. As demand for luxury goods and spices rose, more ships and caravans journeyed to south and central Asia. Much of this trade was carried on through Middle Eastern intermediaries, but, from the twelfth century onward, Europeans played a large and ever-growing role. In all, contacts between East and West flourished as never before. These contacts, so positive for commerce, changed the balance and pattern of infectious diseases. By the end of the twelfth century, Europe's disease pool was stable. Smallpox, measles, malaria, leprosy, and a few other diseases had established a tentative equilibrium within Europe's population. Plague, the greatest epidemic killer, had disappeared. But, in the thirteenth century, climatic changes began to alter the insect and rodent ecology of Eurasia, and Mongol tribesmen began their conquest of central Asia. These factors would combine with the new political, social, and economic forms which were developing in Europe—in part, at least, because of the absence of plague—to forever change the course of Western history.

Chapter 1

The Black Death Ravages Europe

Turning | Points
IN WORLD HISTORY

How the Black Death Entered and Spread Through Europe

Michael W. Dols

Historian Michael W. Dols of California State University at Hayward, here traces the deadly path taken by the Black Death in the 1330s and 1340s. It began in central Asia, he explains, moved westward through the Black Sea region, and then entered the Mediterranean Sea, the coasts and ports of which lay vulnerable to infection. In highlighting the path of the pandemic, Dols cites both Muslim and Christian sources, including the *History* of the fourteenth-century Arabic writer Ibn al-Wardī.

The Black Death almost certainly originated in the Asiatic steppe, where a permanent reservoir of plague infection still exists among the wild rodents of the region: the whole of the Central Asiatic plateau has been called "one huge endemic area." From the steppe, the pandemic spread outward, like the earlier Mongol invasions from this region, to the south and to the west. The Black Death descended on China and India and moved westward to . . . Persia, and finally to the Crimea and the Mediterranean world.

Both the Latin and Arabic sources emphasize the fact that the pandemic was initially accompanied in the Far East by violent ecological changes, such as flooding, famines, and earthquakes. From the Chinese annals, it is clear that the second quarter of the fourteenth century witnessed an unusually large number of damaging environmental disturbances. These natural disasters may have destroyed rodent shelters and food supplies and forced the rodents beyond their normally very restricted habitat into contact with do-

Excerpted from Michael W. Dols, *The Black Death in the Middle East*. Copyright ©1977 by Princeton University Press. Reprinted by permission of Princeton University Press.

mestic rodents and human settlements, carrying the epizootic [animal epidemic] with them. By the end of 1346, it was known, at least in the major Mediterranean seaports, that an unprecedented pestilence was sweeping the Orient. Both the Latin and Arabic authors believed that a corruption of the air, a so-called miasma, had been produced, which was visible in the form of mist or smoke, and was spreading over the land, killing all living things.

Among the Arabic writers on the pandemic, Ibn al-Wardī was an eyewitness to the Black Death in Aleppo and was himself to die of plague in 1349. In his account of the Black Death, he states that the disease had begun in the "land of darkness." This region should be interpreted as inner Asia or Mongolia, and not as China. The pandemic, according to Ibn al-Wardī, had been raging there for fifteen years, which is not an inordinate length of time for the dissemination of the Black Death from its source. . . . If we date the appearance of plague in the Asiatic hinterland from its outbreak in the Crimea in 1346, plague would have reached significant epidemic proportions in Central Asia about the year 1331–1332. . . .

If plague was epidemic in Asia about 1331–1332, as Ibn al-Wardī suggests, it would explain the premature deaths of the Great Khan Jijaghatu Toq-Temür (Wen-Tsong) and his sons. Toq-Temür died on October 2, 1332, at the age of twenty-eight, at Shangtu; his death is chronicled in the Chinese annals among reports of natural disasters that correspond to the Latin tales about the Far East. . . .

Overland Toward the Black Sea

From the history of communicable diseases, we know that epidemics usually follow very closely the commercial trade routes. It is logical, therefore, to investigate the occurrences of plague along the major routes from Asia to the Middle East, in order to establish its probable means of transmission. There were three important routes in the middle of the fourteenth century: (1) the overland route from Mongolia and northern China through Turkestan to the Black Sea region; (2) the combined overland and sea route from India and China through the Indian Ocean and the Persian Gulf to the Fertile Crescent, where the commodities were dispersed among the major commercial centers of the Middle East; and (3) the sea route from the Far East through the Indian Ocean and the Red Sea to Egypt.

Transmission of the Black Death along the second and

The Pestilence Reaches Sicily

This is a small portion of medieval Italian monk Michele da Piazza's account of the arrival of Genoese plague ships in Messina, in northern Sicily.

In October 1347, at about the beginning of the month, twelve Genoese galleys, fleeing from the divine vengeance which Our Lord had sent upon them for their sins, put into the port of Messina. The Genoese carried such a disease in their bodies that if anyone so much as spoke with one of them he was infected with the deadly illness and could not avoid death. The signs of death among the Genoese, and among the Messinese when they came to share the illness with them, were as follows. Breath spread the infection among those speaking together, with one infecting the other, and it seemed as if the victim was struck all at once by the affliction and was, so to speak, shattered by it. This shattering impact, together with the inhaled infection, caused the eruption of a sort of boil, the size of a lentil, on the thigh or arm, which so infected and invaded the body that the victims violently coughed up blood, and after three days' incessant vomiting, for which there was no remedy, they died—and with them died not only anyone who had talked with them, but also anyone who had acquired or touched or laid hands on their belongings.

The people of Messina, realising that the death racing through them was linked with the arrival of the Genoese galleys, expelled the Genoese from the city and harbour with all speed. But the illness remained in the city and subsequently caused enormous mortality.

Michele da Piazza, *Cronaca*, quoted in Rosemary Horrox, ed., *The Black Death*. Manchester, Eng.: Manchester University Press, 1994, p. 36.

third routes appears unlikely. There is no evidence in the Arabic sources of the occurrence of plague in Mesopotamia, Arabia, and Egypt before its appearance in the Crimea or the Mediterranean. . . . Furthermore, these two routes would have carried plague to India beforehand, but there is no concrete evidence that plague infected India before its introduction into the Middle East. . . .

The northern itinerary from the Black Sea to the Asian markets served as the major artery of international trade in the thirteenth and fourteenth centuries, and is the most plausible path of the Black Death. . . .

All the historical sources corroborate the thesis that the Black Death followed this overland route from Central Asia to the Black Sea region, attacking the inhabitants along its path. . . .

From Ibn al-Wardī's *History* we learn that he gathered his information about the course of the Black Death from Muslim merchants returning from the Crimea to Syria. The Black Sea region, as the western terminus of the Asiatic trade route, was an important commercial center for Muslims, as well as for European Christians. The Muslim merchants related to Ibn al-Wardī that the epidemic occurred in October-November 1346, in the land of the Uzbeks—the Golden Horde [the Mongols of what is now southern Russia]—and emptied the villages and towns of their inhabitants. Then it spread to the Crimea and to Byzantium. A *qādī* or Muslim judge in the Crimea, probably in Kaffa, is reported to have said that they counted the dead who were struck by plague, and the number known to them was 85,000. Thus, the account of Ibn al-Wardī concurs with the standard European narrative for the westward dissemination of the pandemic through the Crimea.

From Mongols to Genoese

It is precisely from the Genoese factory at Kaffa that western scholars have traced the transmission of the Black Death to Europe. The basic European source for the westward progress of the pandemic is the account of the transportation of plague by Genoese galleys from the Crimea written by Gabriele de' Mussi. Although the author never left his native town of Piacenza, he must have obtained his information concerning the East—like Ibn al-Wardī—from his compatriots who were trading in the Crimea. The Golden Horde fostered trade with the Genoese and Venetians by allowing the establishment of trading agencies in the Crimea; as was true in Byzantium . . . hostility to the western European states did not prevent active commercial relations. The Crimean trading stations dated from about 1266, when the Mongols ceded land to the Genoese at Kaffa and later at Tana on which to build a consulate and warehouses. However, the Italian merchants had been expelled from Tana in 1343 by the Mongols and were besieged in their fortified city of Kaffa in 1343 and 1345–1346. During the latter siege, plague appeared among the Mongol army, as well as throughout the Golden Horde in 1346. The Kipchak Khan Janibeg (1341–1357) had corpses of his plague-stricken men catapulted over the walls of the city. The Christian defenders hauled the bodies back over the walls and dumped them into the sea. Nevertheless, the infection spread within the city, a fact that de' Mussi attributed to the corrupted air and the poisoned well-water. The Genoese colony was able to put up a stout resistance and compel Janibeg to raise the siege, which was followed by a successful blockade of the Mongol coasts of the Black Sea by the Genoese and Venetian navies. Some of the Genoese, however, fled in their ships to Constantinople and brought plague with them. . . .

Assault on Europe

The Black Death arrived in Sicily early in October, 1347. According to Michael of Piazza, a Franciscan chronicler, it was brought by twelve Genoese galleys, probably from the Crimea or Constantinople, to the port of Messina [in northern Sicily], and radiated out to the rest of the island. The Messinese drove the ships that brought them the disastrous cargo from their port and; in so doing, ensured that it spread more rapidly throughout the western Mediterranean. Following the main trade-routes, the Black Death spread apparently to North Africa by way of Tunis, to Corsica and

Sardinia, to the Balearics, Almería, Valencia, and Barcelona on the Iberian [Spanish] peninsula, and to southern Italy.

The three major centers for the dissemination of the Black Death in southern Europe were Sicily, Genoa, and Venice. In January, 1348, about three months after its arrival in Sicily, plague was introduced into Genoa and Venice. Slightly later, Pisa was struck and served as the point of entry to central and northern Italy. Florence is most closely associated with the Black Death because it was the first great European city to be struck, but also because of the great mortality in the city and the brilliant description of the Black Death by [Italian writer Giovanni] Boccaccio in his preamble to the *Decameron*. The epidemic began to subside by the winter of 1348 in most of Italy but only after having caused an astonishing number of deaths. Despite a multitude of qualifications, Philip Ziegler [a noted scholar of the Black Death] has proposed a decline of a third or slightly more for Italy's total population.

Only a month or two after the arrival of the Black Death on the mainland of Italy, it was brought to Marseilles by a galley that had been expelled from Italy. Driven out, in turn, from Marseilles, the galley contaminated the coast of Languedoc and Spain. The Black Death swept through Marseilles and then began its journey into the hinterland along two main paths. Moving westward, it reached Bordeaux by August, 1348. To the north, it attacked Avignon and Lyons, and reached Paris in June and Burgundy in July and August. The plague in Paris did not abate until the winter of 1349.

From Paris the Black Death advanced northward to the coast in August, 1348. The king of France and the court fled from Paris to Normandy but could not escape; the plague pursued them. By the end of the year, the Black Death had crossed the English Channel and had struck southern England. Having penetrated most of France, it broadened outward, slowly moving through England, Ireland, and Scotland, through Flanders and the Low Countries, and through Germany in 1349.

By June, 1348, the Black Death had crossed the Alps and

had entered Bavaria. It had also travelled through the Balkans into Hungary and Poland, so that central Europe was apparently attacked from three sides. Scandinavia was contaminated from England; plague was reported to have been transmitted by one of the wool ships that sailed from London to Bergen in May, 1349.

With fateful caprice, the Black Death struck the peoples of Europe with varying degrees of intensity, but virtually nowhere was left inviolate. . . . European and Middle Eastern societies shared the same plight. The general degree of depopulation in the West is as uncertain as it is in the Middle East, but the current opinion is that the mortality was at least a quarter of the entire population. It may not be greatly mistaken to estimate that a third of the population of Europe perished from 1348 to 1350.

The Black Death's Grim Death Toll

Johannes Nohl

In this vivid, moving account, the late German scholar Johannes Nohl briefly examines the enormous mortality produced by the onset of the Black Death. He begins by describing some of the various ways that people reacted to the disease, both physically and emotionally, including gruesome scenes of whole families wiped out and decomposing corpses littering the streets. Nohl then goes on to enumerate many of the death tolls for specific regions and cities. Some later scholars have disagreed with his easy acceptance of many of the figures reported by medieval sources, arguing that they are probably exaggerated. Yet even if many of these figures are off by as much as a third, the death toll was still staggering and the scenes of devastation he describes no less real.

"O happy posterity, who will not experience such abysmal woe and will look upon our testimony as a fable." With these words [fourteenth-century Italian poet Francesco] Petrarch concludes his well-known letter in which he describes to a friend the devastation of the town of Florence by the "Black Death." In the years 1345 to 1350 half the population, or, as is maintained by others, one-third of the population, had succumbed to the plague. Two hundred thousand market towns and villages in Europe were completely depopulated, and in the dwellings encumbered with corpses wild beasts took up their abode. Statistics drawn up at the instigation of Pope Clement VI state the number of deaths for the whole world at 42,836,486. . . .

Excerpted from *The Black Death: A Chronicle of the Plague*, compiled by Johannes Nohl, translated by C.H. Clarke (New York: J&J Harper, 1969). Reprinted by permission of Routledge, U.K.

Nowhere Were the Churchyards Sufficient

Reports from different countries and times concerning the suffering caused by the disease vary to an extraordinary extent. Boccaccio makes no reference to pain. Other chroniclers of the fourteenth century report that the sick died within three days gently, as if asleep. Of the children in Germany it is even said that they passed away laughing and singing. In the town of Thornberg the pestilence tormented the people to such a degree that they rent their hands and arms and tore out their hair. In many places in Transylvania they assailed one another in the alleys and streets, and in their frenzy bit and tore each other like dogs and perished miserably.

[Seventeenth-century British writer Daniel] Defoe relates that the plague-boils, when they grew hard and would not burst, caused such terrible pain that they resembled the most exquisite torture, and that many, to escape their torments, threw themselves out of the windows, shot themselves, or took their own lives in some other way. Very frequently the sufferers became demented from horror and pain. Wrapped in their bed-clothes, they rushed to the graves to bury themselves, as they said. In Provence a man climbed to the roof of his house and hurled the tiles into the street. Another executed a mad grotesque dance on the roof till he was shot down by the guard. A third, who for four days had been lying as if dead, awoke suddenly as a prophet, rushed out into the fields and announced the last judgment, exhorted all to repentance, and cursed those who refused to kneel before him. Such scenes naturally augmented the general horror inspired already by the streets and squares encumbered with corpses. The number everywhere was so great that nowhere were the churchyards sufficient. In Erfurt [Germany] in 1350 eleven huge trenches were dug and 12,000 corpses were thrown into them. A memorial tablet was placed there. In St. John's churchyard at Nuremberg [also in Germany] a gravestone from the year 1437 has been preserved:

> Was that not sad and painful to relate,
> I died with thirteen of my house on the same date ? . . .

To ascertain if anyone was still alive in a house the corpse-bearers in many places threw peas or sand against the windows. If no one appeared they entered the dwelling and fetched out the victims of the plague.

In Italy families of seventy persons were completely exterminated, and many heritages passed over to the fourth heir. In Venice alone no less than fifty Patrician [noble] families died out in the year 1348.

The descriptions of the plague from the great cities are particularly heart-rending. . . .

In Marseilles in [the later outbreak of] 1720 the heaps of corpses were so terrible that the streets became impassable. In front of the door of the heroic bishop Belsunzo there were more than one hundred and fifty corpses, half-decomposed and gnawed by dogs. "The stench proceeding from the corpses quickly decaying in the broiling sun is quite indescribable," Belsunzo writes. "A large number of poor sufferers, in fact whole families, are lying in the open air on straw and wretched mattresses. Some are eagerly awaiting the release of death, some are beside themselves from the consuming heat of the poison. And as if the evil by which they have been attacked were not sufficient, they are further exposed to the most acute suffering by the prevailing famine. One's heart is rent at the sight of so many mothers with the corpses of their children beside them, whom they must see die off without being able to help them."

In Vienna also the streets and squares, gardens and vine-yards teemed with the sick and dying. "It has been seen," writes Abraham a Santa-Clara, "that small children were found clinging to the breast of the dead mothers where the innocent little angels could not know that with such drink they were drinking death. It has been seen that when the dead mother was placed on the cart her little daughter tried to accompany her by force, and with a lisping tongue continued to cry, 'Mammy, mammy,' bringing water to the eyes of the rough, hardened corpse-bearers. It has been seen that in the street near the Imperial Market of Himberg a forsaken little baby boy was found together with a goat, which shaggy nurse the little fellow seemed to be beseeching for a drink in baby manner, in the same way as Romulus and Remus were fostered by a wolf. There have been such a quantity of orphans that they were collected by cart-loads and in the hospital formed a small army of children, most of these were besieging the churchyards where they may easily

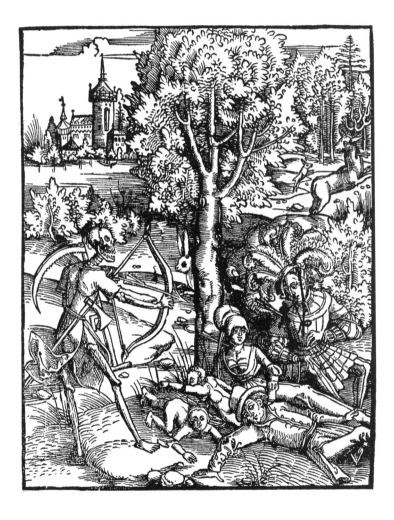

Death, the Grim Reaper, stalks and kills his victims at will in this anonymous sixteenth-century woodcut that first appeared in Geiler von Kaiserperg's "Sermones."

gain admission, such as had recently lost their mothers and were well on the way of returning to the lap of our common mother, earth." It was terrible to see, whole carts full of nobles and citizens—rich and poor, young and old were led through the streets. When the disease had reached its climax it carried off those infected within twenty-four hours. No one remained to cook, to mind the houses. "Such a one is dead, another dying," was all that was said. The seven gates of the city seem insufficient to allow the dead and sick to pass out. Every day there were intercession services; every day the bells tolled. To the loud beating of drums high payment was offered to all who would consent to serve as corpse-bearers and sick-attendants. The town-guard had to round up the unemployed of the servant class, lead several surgeons in chains to the hospitals, and ultimately the prisons had to be thrown open and condemned prisoners set to do the repulsive work.

Ghost Ships and Abandoned Fields

No less harrowing than in the cities is the sight offered by the villages and boroughs. In German chronicles we find the same statements as in [the *Decameron*, by the fourteenth-century Italian writer Giovanni] Boccaccio. Here, too, there is a lack of hands to bury the dead. Here, too, in many places the work of the fields, even the harvest work, had to be suspended, and the cattle strayed from their never-closed byres, abandoned to their own instincts, to return again at night. What the Italian Frari reports from Italy is repeated frequently in the North. "Savage wolves roamed about in packs at night and howled round the walls of the towns. In the villages they did not slake their thirst for human blood by lurking in secret places, as was otherwise their wont, but boldly entered the open houses and tore the little ones from their mothers' sides; indeed they did not only attack children, but even armed men and overcame them. To the contemporaries they seemed no longer wild animals but demons. Other quadrupeds forsook their woods, and in herds approached the vicinity of human habitations, as if aware of the extraordinary conditions. Ravens in innumerable flocks flew over the towns with loud croaking. The kite and the vulture were heard in the air, and other unusual migratory birds appeared. But on the houses the cuckoos and owls alighted and filled the night with their mournful lament. The field-mice had lost all fear and took up their abode among human beings."

Descriptions not to be forgotten are those of ships whose whole crews had been carried off by the plague, and which drifted about as derelicts until cast upon some coast where they brought death and destruction to those who hastened to the rescue: that of the simple goose-girl in the East Pruss-ian estate of Przytullen who, as sole survivor of all the in-habitants, delighted in arraying herself in the dresses and jewels of her dead mistress, and thus in the horrible solitude of the forsaken halls of the manor playing the part of the great lady; that of the young man of Gottersdorf who, hear-ing that the disease had abated, returned to his village and, on entering, met an old man, who greeted him with the words: "I am the only one of the inhabitants left, and now you come. The plague began at the house of one wicked woman, and at the house of another wicked one at the end of the village it ended." That of the parson in Kerenzen on the Wallenstadt Lake who, when all his congregation were dead, inscribed as last survivor his own name in the register of deaths. Of the inhabitants of the chapter house of Bergen in Norway who had fled to the neighbourhood of Tusededal and there began to build a town, "but the disease pursued them there and carried them all off with the exception of one girl. This girl was discovered some years later, but had run wild and was afraid of human beings, and was therefore called the 'rype,' after a wild bird. But when she had been educated for some time all wildness disappeared. She mar-ried, and all the territory in Tusededal which had been marked out for the building of the town was allotted to her and her heirs, who henceforth were known by the name of the 'Rype family.'" Arrid Hoitfeld relates that many marshes were at this time found uncultivated which before the time of the "Black Death" had been ploughed fields, and his book was written three centuries after the epidemic.

The Black Death and the various outbreaks of plague

have found a staggering, graphic expression in "dance of death" pictures and engravings. . . . A "dance of death" representation was possessed practically by every large town. Of those which have been preserved the most celebrated are those of Luebeck, Basle, Berne, Strasbourg, Minden, Paris, Dijon, and London.

The experience incorporated in these graphic representations is the equality of all men in the face of death, an experience of all the greater import as, not only did it shake the foundations of the rigid system of mediæval castes [separation into social classes], but produced the consciousness of the equality of all men before the face of God—that consciousness which led up to the Reformation. If prior to this the higher estimation of the great had been successfully sustained by the . . . innumerable masses said for their souls, this deception failed now that even bishops and prelates frequently remained unburied and their corpses became the food of dogs, and more essential elements than external power and position began to assume the first place in the estimation of men. . . .

Overwhelming Numbers of Dead

The number of victims of the plague in the fourteenth century in Europe is estimated by some to be too low if placed at 25 per cent of the population. The number of victims of [plague outbreaks in] later times with vastly superior hygienic and prophylactic [preventative] conditions must be taken into consideration. Thus in 1467 Moscow mourned the loss of 127,000 victims, Novgorod and district of 230,602, Venice in 1478 of 300,000, Milan 1576, with a population of 200,000 (almost two-thirds of the population are said to have left the town), of 51,000, Berlin in the same year of one-third of its population, Rome of 70,000 in 1591. In Thurgau in 1611 more than half the population died. Milan lost in 1630, 140,000, the Republic of Venice in 1630 and 1631 more than 500,000. In 1630 Cremona was nearly completely depopulated. In Turin there only remained 3,000 persons. In Lorraine, after the plague of 1637, hardly one per cent of the inhabitants was left. Naples lost in 1635,

300,000. London 160,000 in 1665, Vienna in the year 1579 with a population of 210,000, 123,000, Danzic in 1709 in the course of two months 40,000, Marseilles in 1720, 50,000. Toulon in the same year, with a population of 22,000, 13,160; Arles 8,110 from a population of 12,000.

Germany, whose losses for 1348 are estimated at 1,244,434, is one of the countries that suffered least. In Strasbourg there died 16,000; in Erfurt, where there were 1,500 deaths on one single day, at least as many. In Basle 14,000, in Weimar 5,000. The losses were particularly great in the North of Germany. In Pomerania (1356) and Holstein two-thirds of the population died, in Schleswig four-fifths. In Luebeck, which at that time was described as the German Venice, it is reported that of 100 inhabitants not 10 survived. The sum-total is given as 90,000. . . . Chroniclers report in unison that 1,500 died on a single day. In many German districts only 10 survived out of 100 inhabitants, in quite a number only 5. At Vienna between 500 and 700 died daily. On one day it is reported to have been even 960, and on another 1,200. The chronicler of Salzburg writes: "In Vienna there died daily two or three pounds." Now, a pound comprised 240 pfennig or pence, thus the daily number of deaths was between 480 and 720. . . . In the monastery of Marienberg in Vinstgau all the monks died with the exception of four. In the same manner nearly all the monks of the monastery of Dissentis were carried off by the plague. At Meiningen the whole convent of the monastery of the Barefooted Friars died out with the exception of three. Altogether there died of the Order of the Franciscans 124,434.

According to [fourteenth-century French physician] Guy de Chauliac three-quarters of the whole population of France died, according to other reports one-half. In many districts, as, for instance, at Viviers and in Burgundy, nine-tenths died. The thoroughly reliable Gilles de Massis relates of towns where out of 20,000 only 200 survived and of smaller towns where out of 1,500 hardly 100. At Avignon two-thirds were carried off. At Montpelier the losses were so immense that it became necessary to grant citizen rights to Italian merchants in order to repopulate the town.

In Italy half the population died. At Venice 100,000, i.e.

three-quarters of the population. In order to repopulate the town the doge Orseolo invited foreigners to settle at Venice, offering as enticement the acquirement of citizen rights after two years' residence. Of this invitation it seems many Germans availed themselves. In Genoa six-sevenths died. At Bologna and at Padua two-thirds, at Piacenza one-half, at Pisa seven-tenths. The Prince of Carrarra granted an amnesty to all robbers and criminals who would settle in the deserted towns of Padua and Belluno. Scalinger did the same for Verona, which had lost three-quarters of its population. At Siena there died 80,000. At Florence, with a population of roughly 130,000 inhabitants, according to Boccaccio more than 100,000 died. According to Petrarch's report hardly 10 out of 100 survived. From London it was reported that scarcely every tenth man survived. The number of deaths is said to be underestimated at 100,000. At Bristol hardly one-tenth of the population remained. At Norwich out of a population of 70,000 there died 57,374. In England of the clergy alone there died 25,000. From the town of Smolensk in Russia in 1386 there remained only five persons alive. The islands of Cyprus and Iceland are said to have been depopulated to the last inhabitant.

Medieval Medicine's Response to the Black Death

Geoffrey Marks

Having no idea what caused the Black Death, medieval doctors were powerless to stop it and in most cases could not ease the suffering of their patients. This essay by historian Geoffrey Marks, author of several books on the history of medicine, summarizes the primitive medical beliefs of the time and some of the inadequate cures attempted by the baffled and fearful physicians. Some doctors were so fearful, Marks points out, that they refused to treat people or even fled.

In the middle of the fourteenth century France was considered the medical center of the world. The faculty of the Paris College of Physicians was regarded as the final authority. When the Medieval Plague struck, King Philippe de Valois ordered the members of the college to explain the causes of the plague and what should be done about it.

The members announced that they intended to make known the causes of the pestilence "more clearly than could have been done according to the rules and principles of astrology and natural science." They then prepared and presented to the king a declaration that leaned heavily on the movements of the stars and the influence of the sun on nature. This outcome was understandable, their good intentions notwithstanding. Superstition played a major role in medieval life. The not very enlightened doctors of the day were as much slaves to it as others were.

The medical faculty's declaration began by stating that it

was known that the stars had been battling with the sun over India and the neighboring "Great Sea." As a consequence, the rays of the sun had beaten down unmercifully on the sea. The ocean resisted the pull of the sun for twenty-eight days. During this time, "vapors alternatively rose and fell." At length, the fire of the sun's rays fell so powerfully upon the sea that a great portion of its waters was drawn off. The water that was left was so corrupted that the fish in it died. Furthermore, the water not drawn off by the sun was so impure that good water could not be obtained from it. Nor could hail, snow, or dew, which might have brought relief to the land, be produced from it. Instead, the evil waters sent off a vapor which spread itself through the air and reached out to many places on the earth, enveloping them in fog.

Far-fetched and full of myth and superstition as it is, this was the only explanation of how the plague came about that these leading men in medicine could produce. An evil vapor spread through the air and those who breathed it contracted plague.

Of course, there is some basis for their assumption. We have seen that pneumonic plague is transferred from one person to another through the air. We know from the accounts of [contemporary French physician Guy] de Chauliac and others that pneumonic plague was present. But most of the descriptions of the day include the buboes of bubonic plague, which is not transmitted through the air.

Fantastic Cures

If the idea that plague was caused by a vapor that developed when the sun, upset by the stars, dried up the ocean seems fantastic, the proposed cure seems equally fantastic.

The physicians of Paris arrived at this conclusion. The sun and stars caused the plague. Therefore, they would work to get rid of it. They stated without hesitation that it was a function of the stars to protect and heal the human race. In doing so, they worked on and with natural phenomena. In the present case, they would cause the rays of the sun to put forth fire and break through the mist.

Within ten days, the faculty announced, the mist would

be converted into a "stinking deleterious rain" which would continue to fall until July 17. By that date, the air would be purified.

Meantime, all must guard themselves from the effects of the vapor. How? "As soon as this rain announces itself, by thunder or hail, everyone of you should protect himself from the air; and . . . kindle a large fire of vine-wood, green laurel, or other green wood; wormwood and camomile should also be burnt."

This procedure was to be continued until the earth was completely dry again and for three days thereafter. No one was to go out into the fields during this period. A simple diet was to be followed. Poultry and water-fowl, young pork, old beef, and fat meats in general were not to be eaten. The drinking of a broth, seasoned with ground pepper, ginger, and cloves, was highly recommended.

People were advised not to sleep during the daytime. The body was to be kept warmer than usual. But exercise and bathing the body were not considered desirable.

Here was preventive medicine in its crudest form. *If* the plague was the result of evil vapors, large fires could be expected to drive them away before they had been inhaled.

The idea of fires to prevent pestilence actually went back to the fifth century B.C. and Hippocrates. The "father of medicine" firmly believed that epidemics were caused by disturbances in the atmosphere that must be corrected. The Paris physicians were basing their recommendations on good authority.

Green woods were no doubt selected because they would give off an interesting and impressive smoke. Camomile and wormwood were popular medicines of the day. Their inclusion in the wood smoke would do no harm.

Furthermore, if the predicted "stinking, deleterious rain" should arrive on schedule and continue for some time, fires would offer protection from the damp. The fragrant wood smokes would offset the stink of the rain.

The proposed diet seems like a pretty sensible one for people who were to be confined to the hovels they called home for a lengthy period of time. The only instruction that seems wholly meaningless is the one involving no sleep during the daytime.

The complete triviality of this declaration by the greatest medical body of the day is significant. Their advice for the avoidance of plague sounds like a mixture of old wives' tales and witches' brews. Not a word is said about how to cure the plague once it struck or how to ease the suffering of those who contracted it.

These eminent physicians simply did not know. Their position was not unique. Most other doctors shared the general ignorance of their Parisian colleagues.

Gentile da Foligno was a celebrated teacher at Perugia in Italy. He died of plague, "in faithful discharge of his duty," on June 18, 1348. He believed that plague was the result of a "putrid corruption of the blood in the lungs and in the heart, which was occasioned by the pestilential atmosphere, and was forthwith communicated to the whole body." Therefore, to escape the plague, the air must be purified. This was best done by means of large, blazing fires of odoriferous wood. Guy de Chauliac in his turn required the Pope to sit between large fires kindled to purify the air.

Da Foligno set little store by the effects of astrology. However, he was very much alone in holding this viewpoint. Even Guy de Chauliac was convinced that the great mortality had been foreshadowed by a grand conjunction of the three superior planets, Saturn, Jupiter, and Mars, in the sign of Aquarius. This meeting had taken place on March 24, 1345. "Men of science" of the day firmly believed in such portents.

Galeazzo di Santa Sofia of Padua in Italy regarded the influence of the stars as the first cause of plague. A contributory factor was the extensive decomposition of animal and vegetable bodies. He placed special emphasis on the "putrefaction of locusts that had perished in the sea and were again thrown up."

The Church's Influence

There was a major reason why doctors of the day found themselves helpless in the face of the plague. This was control exercised by the Church over medical education and practice.

All universities were under the jurisdiction and domination of the Church. Men of God considered "medical science" of little importance since "its aim was only care of the body and not the mind." This attitude extended beyond a doctor's education.

The first duty of a physician making a house call, the Church said, was to find out if the patient had confessed and received the holy sacrament. If he had not, the doctor was required to obtain his promise to do so. If he refused, he must not treat him.

The Church's position was strengthened by the view held in medieval times that sickness was a manifestation of the wrath of God. It was obviously more important to purge a sick man's soul of his sins than to purge his body of disease.

It was a typical scene in the sickroom for priests to crowd physicians away from the sick bed while they practiced what one writer has described as "pious means of robbery." These practices included appeals to the saints, consecrated candles, holy relics, and Masses. All these services were to be had in exchange for gifts to the Church (or the priest) of money or precious goods. The physician was permitted to try his skill only after the priests had milked the patient. Even then, the priests took credit for the cure, if the physician cured the patient. However, if the physician failed, it was totally his failure.

The church's hold on education produced another hardship for the physician. This was ignorance. The medical education of the day was largely limited to the reading of out-of-date texts. Such comments as the professors might make on these generally followed the party—that is, the Church's—line. Surgery was so weak a sister of whatever medicine might be taught and practiced that early in the fourteenth century the medical faculty of the University of Paris came out "against surgery." It required its entering students to take an oath never to perform a surgical operation. Blood-letting was a common procedure in those days. The Paris faculty required that it be performed by underlings. This led to the emergence of barber-surgeons. In fact, "surgery" paid them so well that many of them gave up shaving and haircutting altogether. Montpellier was by far the most enlightened of contemporary medical schools. But even here there was only one practical lesson in anatomy every two years. . . .

The Theory of Contagion

Doctors believed that the plague had magical origins involving the stars, the atmosphere, and the earth. They believed that a derangement of the humors was a basic cause of all illness. Finally, they believed that plague was highly contagious.

This last miscalculation was the worst because it discouraged doctors from looking further into the means by which bubonic plague is transmitted. The lighting of fires to counteract the impact of the elements certainly did no harm and may have helped in cases of pneumonic plague. The diets which people were cautioned to observe were generally reasonable. Even bloodletting—the medieval cureall—seems to have done at least as much good as it did harm. But the decision that plague was quickly and exclusively passed on through contact with a victim and his possessions prevented doctors from searching for its true roots.

There was ample evidence to support the theory of contagion. Two celebrated contemporary Muhammedan [Muslim] physicians were emphatic on the subject.

"That the evil spreads is evident from observation and experience, it having not yet happened that a well man remained long with a sick one without being attacked by the disease," ibn Khātimah wrote. "Almost as harmful as the air breathed out by the sick, if not entirely so, are the fumes from their bodies, pieces of clothing, beds and linen on which the sick lay, if they are used again. The author has observed . . . that cities which forbade the entry of people from stricken places remained spared as long as possible."

Ibn al-Katîb is quite positive. "The existence of infection stands firm through experience, research, mental perception, autopsy and authentic knowledge of fact, and these are the material proofs," he says.

Simon de Covino was satisfied that once plague "entered

a house scarcely one of those who dwelt in it escaped."

De Chauliac considered plague "so contagious . . . that not only by staying together, but even by looking at one another, people caught it.". . .

To Flee the Only Course?

Since there seemed to be no other answer, flight was the recommendation offered to those that could afford it. Gentile da Foligno who, it will be remembered, himself died of plague, put it this way: "Finally I conclude that to flee . . . is best in this particular pestilence; for this illness is the most poisonous of poisons, and by its spread and blight it affects all."

Da Foligno was echoing the earlier advice of Rhazes, an Arabian physician who lived from 850 to 923 A.D.:

> Three things by which each simple man
> From plague escape and sickness can,
> Start soon, flee far from town or land
> On which the plague has laid its hand,
> Return but late to such a place
> Where pestilence has stayed its pace.

But flight rarely served. Cutthroats, who literally cut throats, infested the highways. In more normal times, the highways were kept relatively safe. The soldiers of the local lords hunted thieves. . . . But now a local lord would find his soldiers reduced by plague from thirty to four. He used the four to guard his own house.

Those who fled and reached their destination without getting their throats cut more often than not included in their company some already carrying the seeds of plague. In any event, plague seemed inevitably to catch up with most of them, however far they flew.

Flight by those who could afford it was not only unavailing. It left a lasting impression on the people of Europe. The poor of Genoa, Florence, Paris, and London saw their "betters" collect their portable riches and take off. The poor too realized that flight was the only defense but few of them could pack up and go. Those who stayed felt deserted and betrayed. Their resentment hastened the decline and disappearance of feudalism.

The only escape doctors could offer their patients was flight. We should not be surprised to find that some followed their own prescription. Flight seems to have been more common from Italian and French towns, where there had been more doctors, than in the north, but there were no hard and fast rules.

Some doctors fled, some stayed. But the motives of those who stayed could be very different. On the one hand, there was a certain Francesco who was asked, when he retired as a health officer after seventeen years service, why he had stayed on in Venice during the plague "when nearly all physicians withdrew on account of fear and terror." He replied quite simply. "I would rather die here than live elsewhere," he said.

On the other hand, the great Guy de Chauliac admitted that he stayed at his post largely because he would have been disgraced if he had quit. "With continual fear, I preserved myself as best I could," he wrote some years later. Nevertheless, having made up his mind to stay, de Chauliac did attend plague patients, he did try to determine the cause of the disease, and he did develop theories for its prevention and cure.

There is evidence of flight on the part of doctors. There is evidence of refusal to treat patients even when offered untold wealth. But there is also evidence that many doctors stayed at their post and died, often heroically. The loss of doctors was great, especially in Italy. Most doctors at Padua died. Piacenza lost twenty of its twenty-four "excellent physicians." Venice was deprived of almost all of its physicians—by flight or death—by early 1348.

And in Montpellier in France, "there was a greater number of physicians than elsewhere, yet scarce one escaped alive."

Anti-Plague Ordinances and Other Social Controls

Ann G. Carmichael

Like doctors and priests, the leaders of individual towns and city-states were largely unable to stop the spread of the Black Death during its outbreaks in the mid-to-late 1300s and early 1400s. Yet a few local leaders did attempt to implement plague controls, ranging from sanitary laws to travel bans, to crude quarantines. And these experiments eventually caught on in other cities, in which such controls often remained almost permanent fixtures. They affected nearly all aspects of society, including the manner of holding funerals, food preparation, and modes of trade and travel. In this excerpt from her book, *Plague and Poor in Renaissance Florence*, Ann G. Carmichael of Indiana University's department of history, examines such plague controls, focusing on their implementation in some northern Italian cities, including Florence, Pistoia, Milan, Mantua, and Venice.

In 1348 Italian communes immediately responded to the threat of epidemic by enforcing traditional sanitary laws. When these failed, they enacted extraordinary crisis measures to minimize social disruption. Finally, they sought in desperation simply to maintain order through the disaster. As much as a century later little had changed in this sequence of responses, despite the frequent recurrence of plague.

Then in the mid-fifteenth century, as if by consensus, Italian legislators decided to isolate plague sufferers by building or designating a lazaretto (pest house). The emphasis on special hospital care shifted from the mere provision of charitable services to isolation of the ill and their contacts. Once hospital isolation of plague sufferers became routine, law-makers phrased their concern for plague control in terms that betrayed their conviction that plague was a contagious disease. By the end of the fifteenth century health boards were widely considered to be necessary bureaucracies in overseeing the enforcement of sanitary law in times of crisis. And, as we have seen, this new legislation had become tinged by the consciousness that poorer persons were more fre-quently the victims and the carriers of plague.

Anti-Plague Ordinances

Pistoia was one of the Tuscan hill towns within the sphere of Florentine influence, a town that provided many immi-grants to Florence. No later than March or April of 1348 plague had penetrated the surrounding district. The Coun-cil of the People met sufficiently regularly until June to record all their efforts to stifle plague's progress. On 23 May 1348 they forbade entrance to the city of any "matter of the illness" (*materia infirmitatis*) from the epidemic reigning in the countryside, referring to both people and goods. Fur-thermore, communication with Lucca and Pisa, towns known to be already infected, was forbidden, except by con-sent of the council. Gatekeepers were assigned to enforce this legislation.

In Pistoia the particulars of epidemic control are much more explicit in the surviving records than they are in Flo-rence. Used clothing, specifically linen rather than wool, was barred from city trade, and articles confiscated from viola-tors were to be publicly burned. Dead bodies had to be placed in wooden caskets "so that no *fetor* [rotten stench] could escape," and had to be buried at least two and one-half arms' lengths deep into the ground. No dead bodies could be transported into the city for burial. Citizens were warned not to associate with the families of victims or enter the house of a victim, and all mourning activities and visits were restricted to "immediate" family. (The deaths of nobles, lawyers, judges, physicians, and other notables could con-tinue to command a greater mourning display.) These crisis measures were set beside a reiteration of traditional legislation: restrictions on the sale of fresh meats, particularly during the summer months, on the slaughter of pigs, on the burning of unused animal flesh, and on the cleaning and tanning of animal hides inside the walls of the city. There is also a hint in the council's proceedings that Pistoians kept a record of all who died.

By June the Council found it "almost impossible" to assemble a quorum of elders and to continue official provisions. Records disappeared after 27 June, following attempts to revise the number needed for passing new legislation. The last known ordinances before 27 June were directed toward sanitation and funeral display. No bell ringing should accompany burial of the dead, no funeral processions could follow the deceased to the church. Mourning was restricted to immediate family and relatives on the mother's side only. Sixteen men for each district were hired to extract the dead from their houses and deposit them at the church for burial. The public porters would be paid from communal funds so long as they gave written notification of the burial, cosigned by the priest, monk, or hospital rector at the burial ground. The council still enjoined "good men" to carry and bury the poor without remuneration. The number of candles burned for the dead would be severely limited, and churches were to curtail the use of torches.

Elsewhere in Tuscany, Luccans proscribed [forbade] travelers from Genoa and Catalonia as early as 14 January 1348—though to no avail. The Perugians, according to a local chronicler, even boasted a team of physicians dissecting plague victims to ascertain the causes of plague. No record of public health measures in Perugia survives from 1348, but a chronicler noted that physicians counseled their private patients to be careful of diet and to ingest prophylactic medicines (especially purgatives) that would prepare the body to withstand corrupt air.

Venetian officials, far removed from Tuscany, also created a special health board to deal with the Black Death. A three-man commission concentrated their efforts on sanitation just as had Florentines. With even more reason than the Pistoians had, they worried about health measures in burial. New cemeteries had to be consecrated quickly to receive all the bodies; boatmen were needed to transport them. Burial pits needed to be dug to a minimum depth of five feet. As in Lucca and Pisa, ill foreigners were quickly perceived to be a source of infection, especially when the epidemic began to worsen. Incarcerating travelers and burning their goods, including the boats carrying them, became possible penalties for infraction of the new rules. . . .

Some Crude Quarantines

Real changes in sanitary legislation began with the initiation of quarantine, but that measure was not used on the Italian mainland before the fifteenth century. Venice's small Adriatic colony, Ragusa (now Dubrovnik), adopted in 1377 a thirty-day period of isolating travelers and their goods. The isolation applied to all travelers, not just those coming from a locale where plague raged. Thus the quarantine isolated healthy individuals and their goods in order to halt the extension of infection. The original quarantine was not motivated by an early appeal to contagion as an explanation of the spread of disease. It was instead a passive waiting and watching for a hidden epidemic. Legislators fully expected the air to become locally infected if plague was incubating aboard ship. The Ragusans, utterly dependent on sea trade and having little commerce with the mainland, could be reasonably sure that plague was transported to the city from outside. No other obvious source of infection existed. In the original quarantine, no traveler's good health was taken for granted and no provisions were made for the isolation of plague stricken individuals once plague appeared. The original legislation contained no explicit defense of a contagion theory; even in Ragusa measures to isolate the ill did not appear until the mid-fifteenth century.

The external origin of plague was less apparent to inhabitants of inland cities or of ports having extensive communication with inland hinterlands than it was to the Ragusans. Most cities did not develop anything like a quarantine before the fifteenth century. Two exceptions are worth mentioning,

for they show that a single, powerful ruler could enforce unpopular legislation isolating well individuals. In both cases,
however, the rulers were convinced that plague was contagious and could be carried by healthy individuals who traveled from a region where plague raged. Thus they did not
defend the quarantine as a passive defense against infection.
Not surprisingly, in both Milan and Mantua the ruler's belief in plague contagion dictated the adoption of additional
measures to isolate those suffering from plague as well.

Within the space of a few months, and several years before Ragusa's quarantine, Bernabò Visconti of Milan and
Ludovico Gonzaga of Mantua took unusual steps to defend
these two cities from epidemic. The Milanese proscription
was earlier (17 January 1374) and is fairly well known. Bernabò Visconti wrote to an official in Reggio in Emilia the
measures that he thought were most useful to control plague
in the city. Priests would view the ill in their parishes and notify inquisitors of the nature of the disease. The stricken
would be sent outside the city walls. All of these provisions
operated on the basic presupposition that plague was a contagious disease, and so it was treated just as leprosy had been
in the preceding centuries. Visconti's ordinance even admits
that he wished to preserve Milan and its territory "from contagious maladies."

Ludovico Gonzaga decreed sometime in 1374 that any
Mantuan who passed through a place where the great mortality raged could not then reenter the city. Those who violated the new law risked death. . . . The vicars, themselves
under threat of death if they disobeyed, were additionally
obliged to enforce this legislation, burning transgressors'
goods and houses. There was no specific mention of a fixed
period of isolation, as there was in the Ragusan quarantine,
but the Milanese and Mantuan examples did apply to all
citizens.

The early Mantuan and Milanese examples suggest that
tyrants had uncontested, unqualified authority over their
cities. Neither ruler apparently listened to conflicting medical
opinions, and neither apparently considered astrological explanations for the appearance of plague. Gonzaga and Visconti

had the power to do something that was politically and economically unpopular and that violated medical counsel as well.

Travel Bans and Crisis Management

By 1400 anyone passing through Mantuan territory needed official license (a *boletino*) to travel during plague times. As early as 1374 Bernabò Visconti had designated official guards to prohibit anyone from a plague region entering Milan. His successor, Giangaleazzo Visconti, exercised an even greater power in extending preventive plague bans. By August 1397, Giangaleazzo banned all travelers coming from plague-ridden Belluno. As the great plague of 1400 approached, the proscriptions escalated.

Giangaleazzo appointed one trusted official to coordinate all his bans, proclamations, and plague-relief measures. First, all the towns in Visconti domain were proscribed as they became plague infected. Each town had to obey trade and travel restrictions and actively provide assistance to its infected citizens. . . . Giangaleazzo augmented preventive plague measures to include the fumigation of houses where plague had occurred. He was also clearly unwilling to accept halfway quarantine measures as citizens had done. He ordered that "suspects" or survivors of plague households should be transported out of the city to houses (*mansiones*) of recovery, and he severely restricted fairs and festivals that would increase the association of the sick and healthy.

Once plague broke out in Milan, however, most of the duke's provisions aimed only at managing the crisis. In 1399 Giangaleazzo ordered that Milan's city gates be closed during the plague assault, as he frequently did when war made Milan vulnerable to foreign invasion, but there is no evidence that he allowed guards to protect the property of absentee citizens. He tried to ensure a supply of foodstuffs, since he thought that famine could lead to further plague. He ordered that the sick be carried to hospitals, and when the plague worsened he forbade the well to leave, demanding that they assume the jobs of the sick and dead. Wagons to collect the poor and transport them to hospitals had been employed since 1396, and they were used extensively during the plague. The sick lived in fear of the rattle of carriages.

Other Cities Adopt Plague Controls

All the Visconti legislation was based on the ruler's belief in the contagious spread of plague. It was not a program widely imitated in 1400 or in the generation that followed because it was costly and difficult to enforce, but more importantly because most northern Italians in 1400 did not believe in the contagiousness of plague. A contagion theory acceptable to university-trained physicians needed to explain precisely what could be transmitted by contact. Even [the great ancient Greek physician] Galen had ultimately rejected the notion of invisible particles or substances passed from one body to another, in favor of a generalized corruption of ambient air that could corrupt body humors. Giangaleazzo died of a "pestilential fever" in 1402, and his successor, Gian Maria Visconti, continued to enforce his program of plague control. However, the measures were abandoned by the time of the plague of 1406 in Milan. There was no comparable legislation to fight plague in Milan until 1424, and then the provisions did not stem from the Visconti Duke or his personal secretaries. In the generation between 1424 and mid-century, widespread interest in controlling the spread of plague emerged throughout northern Italy.

Under Filippo Maria Visconti's rule (1412–47) official bans began to appear from the "Vicar of Provisions," the "Twelve of Provision," and the "Commissioner of Health." In other words, the plague controls in the fifteenth century became separated institutionally from the duke and his retinue. Consequently the commission turned more attention to Milan's needs. It prohibited change of habitation within the city during a plague, as well as the movement of household goods; houses where someone had died of plague had to be aired out thoroughly. . . .

The Perugians proclaimed in 1424 that no citizen could lodge a foreigner coming from a place suspected of being plague ridden. In mid-July 1424, the council of Udine banned all travelers from infected places, except those who had the express license of the council. The Venetian senate even sent out warnings to galley captains to avoid places infected with plague. Similarly in Mantua the Gonzaga lord issued the same sort of plague restrictions many city-states were finding necessary in 1428: No one could harbor an outsider traveling from a plague site; no citizen could leave and return home if he traveled to a plague region; and no one from a plague-infected house could move elsewhere. . . .

In sum, mid-fifteenth-century bans on travel and trade from plague regions were the first real innovations for inland cities and towns. These measures are based upon the basic quarantine idea (i.e., segregating persons and merchandise to prevent the progress of plague into a territory), but the restrictions were limited to those people and goods that have passed through a plague region. True maritime quarantine was not feasible for inland cities and towns. The measures also may have provided a network of information about safe regions and cities.

Atoning for Humanity's Sins: The Flagellants

Otto Friedrich

Because the Black Death appeared in the eyes of most people of the fourteenth century to be a punishment sent by God, it seemed logical that fervent appeals to God might alleviate the crisis. Some of the most fanatically devout, who came to be known as the flagellants, took this idea to its extreme. They decided that severe public displays of self-punishment would show God that humanity had seen the error of its sinful ways and would solicit His forgiveness. In this excerpt from his acclaimed book, *The End of the World: A History*, journalist/historian Otto Friedrich traces the early background of the flagellants and describes in detail their bizarre ceremonies and tactics. He also tells how Pope Clement VI, who had recently moved his papal court from Rome to Avignon in southern France, at first gave the flagellants his blessing; but later, perceiving them as a distinct threat to the Church's authority, he denounced them.

If mankind was guilty of having provoked this divine punishment, then mankind must expiate [atone for] its guilt, and the convulsive movement toward that expiation suddenly erupted in Germany. Religious flagellation had its precedents, of course. The anchorites of the early Christian era made their sufferings a form of worship, and the tradition flickered on in various monastic communities. The first public demonstration of self-scourging as a means of appeasing divine wrath seems to have been led by a Perugian hermit named Raniero in 1260, and the strange practice soon spread all over Italy.

Excerpted from Otto Friedrich, *The End of the World: A History* (New York: Fromm International, 1986). Copyright ©1982 by Otto Friedrich. Reprinted by permission of the Estate of Otto Friedrich and the Aaron Priest Literary Agency, New York.

73

That too had been a time of famine and pestilence. It had also been the year when, according to the widely circulated prophecies of Joachim of Fiore, the world was destined to pass through the reign of Antichrist and enter its third and last great epoch, the Age of the Holy Spirit. The relatively uneventful passage of the apocalyptic year dulled the fever of anticipation, but flagellation survived north of the Alps as a somewhat furtive and almost heretical ritual. With the coming of the plague, it was furtive no longer.

Marching Barefoot and Singing Hymns

The Brotherhood of the Flagellants first appeared in Dresden, in Lent of 1349, then in Lübeck, Hamburg, Magdeburg, all over central Europe. They seemed to have no single leader, but they subscribed to a strict discipline, and their processions often numbered as many as five thousand, sometimes more. They marched two by two, the men separated from the women, and as this serpentine parade of penitence neared a town the church bells would sound, and all the citizens would gather to watch the spectacle. There were elements of pure theater in these demonstrations, and also of tormented eroticism, but most citizens regarded the flagellants, at least in the early days, much as the flagellants regarded themselves, as lambs of God bearing the sins of the earth. A flagellant who undertook to whip himself and implore God's mercy on behalf of less courageous sinners could only be viewed as a hero, rather as modern observers might view some dedicated doctor who entered a plague-ridden slum to bring medicine to infected victims.

They marched barefoot. They wore ankle-length white linen underclothing and cloaks of penitential black, and on their cloaks they had sewn red crosses. Their heads were covered with hoods, surmounted by gray felt hats. They carried banners of purple velvet, also bearing the emblem of the cross. They never spoke, but they sang almost incessantly:

"Our journey's done in the holy name.
Christ Himself to Jerusalem came.
His cross He bore in His holy hand,
Help us, Savior of all the land. . . ."

Twice every day and once every night, they performed their rituals of expiation, sometimes in a church, sometimes in a crowded market place. They took off everything except their white underclothes, then marched in a circle, beating themselves until they bled, and singing.

"Come here for penance good and well,
Thus we escape from burning hell. . . ."

They knelt down and stretched out their arms as if being crucified and then fell to the ground. They assumed different positions of supplication, representing different sins for which they were doing penance, real or symbolic. The murderer lay on his back, the adulterer on his stomach, the perjurer on one side with three fingers stretched above his head. Two elected masters passed among the penitents, delivering one blow to each and offering absolution:

"By Mary's honor free from stain,
Arise and do not sin again."

In Christ's Name

The flagellants arose, but only to resume scourging themselves for the sins of those citizens who crowded around and groaned at their ordeal. These were not merely symbolic demonstrations. "Each scourge," according to one chronicler, Heinrich of Herford, "was a kind of stick from which three tails with large knots hung down. Through the knots were thrust iron spikes as sharp as needles, which penetrated about the length of a grain of wheat or a little more beyond the knots. With such scourges they beat themselves on their naked bodies so that they became swollen and blue, and blood ran down to the ground and spattered the walls of the churches in which they scourged themselves. Occasionally they drove the spikes so deep into the flesh that they could only be pulled out by a second wrench."

When the scourging was done, the flagellants once again chanted their hymn, "Our journey's done in the holy name . . ." Then their master led them to the cross, where they fell to their knees while the master intoned the words

"Hail Mary, sweet Mother Mary, have pity upon thy miserable Christendom." And again: "Hail Mary!" And again: "Hail Mary, rose in the kingdom of heaven, have mercy upon us and upon all faithful souls." After this series of incantations, the master read aloud the "flagellant sermon," a thirteenth-century document that purported to be a letter written by Jesus Christ on a marble tablet. This tablet was said to have fallen from heaven onto the altar of the Church of the Holy Sepulcher in Jerusalem.

"O ye children of men, ye of little faith," Christ's letter began, "ye have not believed My words. . . . Therefore did I send against you the Saracens and heathen people, who have spilt your blood and led you into bondage. Further, I have sent tribulation upon you, earthquake, famine, beasts; serpents, mice and locusts; hail, lightning and thunder, and severe disease; but ye closed your ears and would not hearken to My voice. . . . I thought to exterminate you from the earth, but My host of angels, falling at My feet, besought Me to turn away wrath, and I have shown mercy. . . . I swear to you by My raised hand, if ye are not converted and observe My commandments, My wrath will be vented on you. . . . I will send upon you wild beasts such as have never been seen and wild birds, I will convert the light of the sun into darkness so that one may slaughter the other, and there will be great wailing, and I will smother your souls with smoke, send terrible peoples against you, who will not spare you, and devastate your land, all because ye have not kept my Sabbath."

A Yearning for Suffering

The flagellants began as a kind of monastic order, a kind of crusade. They pledged themselves to these wanderings for thirty-three and a half days, a symbolic re-creation of Christ's years of wandering on this earth. They also pledged themselves to absolute obedience in a search for sanctity. "We undertake to avoid every opportunity of doing evil to others to the best of our ability," according to one version of the Statutes of the Order of Flagellants preserved in the chronicle of Hugo von Reutlingen, "to repent of all sins of which we are conscious and to make a general confession thereof; to dispose by legal will and testament of all legally acquired possessions; . . . to pay all debts and restore all wrongfully acquired possessions; to live in peace, to improve our lives and show restraint toward others; to stake life and limb, goods and chattels for the defense and preservation of the rights of the Holy Church . . ."

A Bloody Procession

This short description of the actions of a band of flagellants is by the medieval English chronicler Robert of Avesbury.

In that same year of 1349, about Michaelmas [29 September], more than 120 men, for the most part from Zeeland or Holland, arrived in London from Flanders. These went barefoot in procession twice a day in the sight of the people, sometimes in St Paul's church and sometimes elsewhere in the city, their bodies naked except for a linen cloth from loins to ankle. Each wore a hood painted with a red cross at front and back and carried in his right hand a whip with three thongs. Each thong had a knot in it, with something sharp, like a needle, stuck through the middle of the knot so that it stuck out on each side, and as they walked one after the other they struck themselves with these whips on their naked, bloody bodies; four of them singing in their own tongue and the rest answering in the manner of the Christian litany. Three times in each procession they would all prostrate themselves on the ground, with their arms outstretched in the shape of a cross. Still singing, and beginning with the man at the end, each in turn would step over the others, lashing the man beneath him once with his whip, until all of those lying down had gone through the same ritual. Then each one put on his usual clothes and, always with their hoods on their heads and carrying their whips, they departed to their lodgings. It was said that they performed a similar penance every night.

Quoted in Rosemary Horrox, ed., *The Black Death*. Manchester, Eng.: Manchester University Press, 1994, pp. 153–54.

Anyone joining this crusade had to have the permission of husband or wife, had to bring enough money to pay for bread and shelter (about ten pennies per day), had to agree to a life of absolute austerity, no bed at night, only a layer of straw, no bathing, no shaving, no washing of the head, no change of clothing, no conversation with any member of the opposite sex. And endless prayer: three Paternosters and three Ave Marias on arising in the morning, five more before and after each meal, and five more before sleep, and five during each scourging. . . .

This yearning for suffering, for wild excess, for passion, for religious experience beyond anything taught or advocated by the church, caused both the cancerous growth and the eventual suppression of the flagellants. Despite their talk of preserving the rights of the church, the flagellants were a lay movement, and by threatening implication an anticlerical movement. The masters of the march were laymen, and their chants were the first vernacular [non-Latin] hymns that the Germans had ever heard. And though the flagellants conducted their rituals in churches, they did so more or less by force, as riotous invaders whom the parish priests were too frightened to resist. Two Dominicans who tried to halt a flagellant ritual near Moisson were stoned by the worshipers, one of them to death.

These demonstrations soon acquired a radical political coloring. Many terrified Germans were living in expectation of an imminent restoration of the Emperor Frederick II, who had been widely regarded a century earlier as the man destined to become the universal ruler and to chastise the church on the eve of the apocalypse. Many other citizens simply wanted to vent their anxiety and anger against the clergy, the rich, the established authorities. So thousands of people flocked to the flagellant movement, and it spread outward into Bohemia, Hungary, Flanders. In the summer of 1349, a procession of flagellants at Constance was said to number 42,000, and a march through Brabant at Christmas was reputed to total more than eighty thousand. In Strasbourg, new troops of flagellants kept arriving to stage their rituals every week for six months.

Vanishing like "Night Phantoms"

The church could hardly help being alarmed. When Pope Clement first heard of the flagellants, he agreed to attend a parade in which two thousand of them marched through Avignon. He even blessed them. But he soon began to receive disturbing reports from his bishops that these blood-stained penitents were undertaking to perform the sacramental functions of the church itself. And in defending their actions, the flagellants spoke with the voice of heresy. . . . "When the flagellants were asked," according to one account, "'Why do ye preach, having received no mission . . . ?' they replied, turning the tables, 'Who, then, gave you a mission, and how do ye know that ye consecrate the body of Christ or that what ye preach is the true Gospel?' If they were told that the church could not err as it was guided by the Holy Ghost, then they replied that they received their instruction and mission most directly from the Lord and the spirit of the Lord." The itinerant flagellant masters began to perform sacraments, hear confessions, grant forgiveness. They claimed, in some instances, to be able to cast out evil spirits and to heal the sick. Their bloodstained rags were preserved and venerated as holy relics. In Strasbourg, they tried and failed to bring a dead child back to life. They claimed, more and more insistently, that their movement must last thirty-three and a half years, and then end in the Second Coming. And people believed them. "Many persons, and even young children, were soon bidding farewell to the world," according to one chronicle, "some with prayers, others with praises on their lips."

The established powers have always resisted such passions. King Philip of France forbade all flagellants to enter his kingdom, and provincial authorities appealed to the theologians of the Sorbonne [a renowned university in Paris] for an authoritative opinion on this outbreak of self-mortification. The Sorbonne disapproved, and expressed its disapproval by sending a Flemish monk named Jean da Fayt to Avignon to argue the case before Clement. From Germany itself, Emperor Charles IV petitioned the Pope for counsel. The Pope understood; his sympathy for these zealots had been a mistake. In a papal bull issued in October of 1349, Clement denounced the flagellants and banished them from all Christian communities. "Already," he declared, "flagellants under pretense of piety have spilled the blood of Jews, which Christian charity preserves and protects, and frequently also the blood of Christians, and, when opportunity offered, they have stolen the property of the clergy and laity and have arrogated to themselves the legal authority of their superiors. . . . We therefore command our archbishops and suffragans that in their dioceses they declare in our name as godless and forbidden all societies, meetings, uses and statutes of the so-called flagellants, which we at the advice of our brethren have condemned . . ."

It was so ordered and so carried out. Although popular protests prevented the reading of the bull in some towns, the united opposition of the Pope, the Emperor, and the King of France was invincible. The chroniclers' accounts of flagellant processions fade into passing mentions of flagellants hanged in Westphalia, burned in Breslau, beheaded in Trier. Some of them appeared in Rome during the Jubilee of 1350 to expiate their heresy by being lashed before the altar of Saint Peter, but most of them simply disappeared into the countryside, "vanishing as suddenly as they had come," in the words of one chronicler, "like night phantoms or mocking ghosts."

The Black Death Blamed on the Jews

Barbara W. Tuchman

Greatly compounding the human tragedy of mass death by the Black Death was the persecution and mass murder of Jews during the disease's major outbreak in the mid-fourteenth century. In this dramatic tract from her widely read and acclaimed study of the period, two-time Pulitzer Prize-winning historian Barbara W. Tuchman summarizes the Jews' plight. She begins with a detailed examination of the growth of anti-Semitic feelings among European Christians. Then she chronicles the widely-believed charges that the pestilence was caused by Jews poisoning Christian water sources and the horrendous killings and other abuses perpetrated by Christians on Jews in retaliation for this imaginary crime.

St. Roch, credited with special healing powers, who had died in 1327, was the particular saint associated with the plague. Inheriting wealth as a young man, as had St. Francis, he had distributed it to the poor and to hospitals, and while returning from a pilgrimage to Rome had encountered an epidemic and stayed to help the sick. Catching the malady himself, he retreated to die alone in the woods, where a dog brought him bread each day. "In these sad times," says his legend, "when reality was so somber and men so hard, people ascribed pity to animals." St. Roch recovered and, on appearing in rags as a beggar, was thought to be a spy and thrown into jail, where he died, filling the cell with a strange light. As his story spread and sainthood was conferred, it was believed that God would cure of the plague anyone who invoked his name. When this failed to occur, it enhanced the belief that, men having grown too wicked, God indeed intended their end. As [the medieval English poet William] Langland wrote,

> God is deaf now-a-days and deigneth not hear us,
> And prayers have no power the Plague to stay.

In a terrible reversal, St. Roch and other saints now came to be considered a source of the plague, as instruments of God's wrath. "In the time of that great mortality in the year of our Lord 1348," wrote a professor of law named Bartolus of Sassoferrato, "the hostility of God was stronger than the hostility of man." But he was wrong.

Origins of Anti-Jewish Hatred

The hostility of man proved itself against the Jews. On charges that they were poisoning the wells, with intent "to kill and destroy the whole of Christendom and have lordship over all the world," the lynchings began in the spring of 1348 on the heels of the first plague deaths. The first attacks occurred in Narbonne and Carcassonne, where Jews were dragged from their houses and thrown into bonfires. While Divine punishment was accepted as the plague's source, people in their misery still looked for a human agent upon whom to vent the hostility that could not be vented on God. The Jew, as the eternal stranger, was the most obvious target. He was the outsider who had separated himself by choice from the Christian world, whom Christians for centuries had been taught to hate, who was regarded as imbued with unsleeping malevolence against all Christians. Living in a distinct group of his own kind in a particular street or quarter, he was also the most feasible target, with property to loot as a further inducement.

The accusation of well-poisoning was as old as the plague of Athens, when it had been applied to the Spartans, and as recent as the epidemics of 1320–21, when it had been applied to the lepers. At that time the lepers were believed to have acted at the instigation of the Jews and the Moslem King of Granada, in a great conspiracy of outcasts to destroy

Christians. Hundreds were rounded up and burned throughout France in 1322 and the Jews heavily punished by an official fine and unofficial attacks. When the plague came, the
charge was instantly revived against the Jews:

> . . . rivers and fountains
> That were clear and clean
> They poisoned in many places . . .

wrote the French court poet Guillaume de Machaut.

The antagonism had ancient roots. The Jew had become
the object of popular animosity because the early Church,
as an offshoot of Judaism striving to replace the parent, had
to make him so. His rejection of Christ as Saviour and his
dogged refusal to accept the new law of the Gospel in place
of the Mosaic law made the Jew a perpetual insult to the
newly established Church, a danger who must be kept distinct and apart from the Christian community. This was the
purpose of the edicts depriving Jews of their civil rights issued by the early Church Councils in the 4th century as
soon as Christianity became the state religion. Separation
was a two-way street, since, to the Jews, Christianity was at
first a dissident sect, then an apostasy with which they
wanted no contact.

The theory, emotions, and justifications of anti-Semitism
were laid at that time—in the canon law codified by the
Councils; in the tirades of St. John Chrysostom, Patriarch of
Antioch, who denounced the Jews as Christ-killers; in the
judgment of St. Augustine, who declared the Jews to be "outcasts" for failing to accept redemption by Christ. The Jews'
dispersion was regarded as their punishment for unbelief.

The period of active assault began with the age of the crusades, when all Europe's intramural antagonisms were gathered into one bolt aimed at the infidel. On the theory that
the "infidel at home" should likewise be exterminated, massacres of Jewish communities marked the crusaders' march
to Palestine. The capture of the Holy Sepulcher by the
Moslems was blamed on "the wickedness of the Jews," and
the cry "HEP! HEP!" for *Hierosolyma est Perdita* (Jerusalem is
lost) became the call for murder. What man victimizes he

fears; thus, the Jews were pictured as fiends filled with hatred of the human race, which they secretly intended to destroy.

Merciless Monsters?

The question whether Jews had certain human rights, under the general proposition that God created the world for all men including infidels, was given different answers by different thinkers. Officially the Church conceded some rights: that Jews should not be condemned without trial, their synagogues and cemeteries should not be profaned, their property not be robbed with impunity. In practice this meant little because, as non-citizens of the universal Christian state, Jews were not allowed to bring charges against Christians, nor was Jewish testimony allowed to prevail over that of Christians. Their legal status was that of serfs of the king, though without reciprocal obligations on the part of the overlord. The doctrine that Jews were doomed to perpetual servitude as Christ-killers was announced by Pope Innocent III in 1205 and led Thomas Aquinas to conclude with relentless logic that "since Jews are the slaves of the Church, she can dispose of their possessions." Legally, politically, and physically, they were totally vulnerable.

They maintained a place in society because as moneylenders they performed a role essential to the kings' continuous need of money. Excluded by the guilds from crafts and trades, they had been pushed into petty commerce and moneylending although theoretically barred from dealing with Christians. Theory, however, bends to convenience, and Jews provided Christians with a way around their self-imposed ban on using money to make money.

Since they were damned anyway, they were permitted to lend at interest rates of 20 percent and more, of which the royal treasury took the major share. The increment to the crown was in fact a form of indirect taxation; as its instruments, the Jews absorbed an added measure of popular hate. They lived entirely dependent upon the king's protection, subject to confiscations and expulsions and the hazards of royal favor. Nobles and prelates followed the royal example, entrusting money to the Jews for lending and taking most of the profits, while deflecting popular resentment upon the agent. To the common man the Jews were not only Christ-killers but rapacious, merciless monsters, symbols of the new force of money that was changing old ways and dissolving old ties.

As commerce swelled in the 12th and 13th centuries, increasing the flow of money, the Jews' position deteriorated in proportion as they were less needed. They could not deal in the great sums that Christian banking houses like the Bardi of Florence could command. Kings and princes requiring ever larger amounts now turned to the Lombards and wealthy merchants for loans and relaxed their protection of the Jews or, when in need of hard cash, decreed their expulsion while confiscating their property and the debts owed to them. At the same time, with the advent of the Inquisition in the 13th century, religious intolerance waxed, leading to the charge of ritual murder against the Jews and the enforced wearing of a distinctive badge.

The belief that Jews performed ritual murder of Christian victims, supposedly from a compulsion to re-enact the Crucifixion, began in the 12th century and developed into the belief that they held secret rites to desecrate the host. Promoted by popular preachers, a mythology of blood grew in a mirror image of the Christian ritual of drinking the blood of the Saviour. Jews were believed to kidnap and torture Christian children, whose blood they drank for a variety of sinister purposes ranging from sadism and sorcery to the need, as unnatural beings, for Christian blood to give them a human appearance. Though bitterly refuted by the rabbis and condemned by emperor and pope, the blood libel took possession of the popular mind most rabidly in Germany, where the well-poisoning charge too had originated in the 12th century. The blood libel formed the subject of Chaucer's tale of a child martyr told by the Prioresse [in the *Canterbury Tales*] and was the ground on which many Jews were charged, tried, and burned at the stake.

Mounting Restrictions Against Jews

Under the zeal of St. Louis, whose life's object was the greater glory and fulfillment of Christian doctrine, Jewish life in France was narrowed and harassed by mounting restrictions. The famous trial of the Talmud [collection of ancient Jewish holy writings] for heresy and blasphemy took place in Paris in 1240 during his reign, ending in foreordained conviction and burning of 24 cartloads of Talmudic works. . . .

Throughout the century the Church multiplied decrees designed to isolate Jews from Christian society, on the theory that contact with them brought the Christian faith into disrepute. Jews were forbidden to employ Christians as servants, to serve as doctors to Christians, to intermarry, to sell flour, bread, wine, oil, shoes, or any article of clothing to Christians, to deliver or receive goods, to build new synagogues, to hold or claim land for non-payment of mortgage. The occupations from which guild rules barred them included weaving, metalworking, mining, tailoring, shoemaking, goldsmithing, baking, milling, carpentry. To mark their separation, Innocent III in 1215 decreed the wearing of a badge, usually in the form of a wheel or circular patch of yellow felt, said to represent a piece of money. Sometimes green or red-and-white, it was worn by both sexes beginning between the ages of seven and fourteen. In its struggle against all heresy and dissent, the 13th century Church imposed the same badge on Moslems, on convicted heretics, and, by some quirk in doctrine, on prostitutes. A hat with a point rather like a horn, said to represent the Devil, was later added further to distinguish the Jews.

Expulsions and persecutions were marked by one constant factor—seizure of Jewish property. As the chronicler William of Newburgh wrote of the massacre of York in 1190, the slaughter was less the work of religious zeal than of bold and covetous men who wrought "the business of their own greed." The motive was the same for official expulsion by towns or kings. When the Jews drifted back to resettle in villages, market towns and particularly in cities, they continued in moneylending and retail trade, kept pawnshops, found an occupation as gravediggers, and lived close together in a narrow Jewish quarter for mutual protection. In [the French region of] Provence, drawing on their contact with the Arabs of Spain and North Africa, they were scholars and sought-after physicians. But the vigorous inner life of their earlier communities had faded. In an excitable period they lived on the edge of assault that was always imminent. It was understood that the Church could "justly ordain war upon them" as enemies of Christendom.

Some Attempts to Protect the Jews

In the torment of the plague it was easy to credit Jewish malevolence with poisoning the wells. In 1348 Clement VI issued a Bull prohibiting the killing, looting, or forcible conversion of Jews without trial, which halted the attacks in Avignon and the Papal States but was ignored as the rage swept northward. Authorities in most places tried at first to protect the Jews, but succumbed to popular pressure, not without an eye to potential forfeit of Jewish property.

In Savoy, where the first formal trials were held in September 1348, the Jews' property was confiscated while they remained in prison pending investigation of charges. Composed from confessions extracted by torture according to the usual medieval method, the charges drew a picture of an international Jewish conspiracy emanating from Spain, with messengers from Toledo carrying poison in little packets or in a "narrow stitched leather bag." The messengers allegedly brought rabbinical instructions for sprinkling the poison in wells and springs, and consulted with their co-religionists in secret meetings. Duly found guilty, the accused were condemned to death. Eleven Jews were burned alive and the rest subjected to a tax of 160 florins every month over the next six years for permission to remain in Savoy.

The confessions obtained in Savoy, distributed by letter from town to town, formed the basis for a wave of accusations and attacks throughout Alsace, Switzerland, and Germany. At a meeting of representatives of Alsatian towns, the oligarchy of Strasbourg attempted to refute the charges but were overwhelmed by the majority demanding reprisal and expulsion. The persecutions of the Black Death were not all spontaneous outbursts but action seriously discussed beforehand.

Again Pope Clement attempted to check the hysteria in a Bull of September 1348 in which he said that Christians who imputed the pestilence to the Jews had been "seduced by that liar, the Devil," and that the charge of well-poisoning and ensuing massacres were a "horrible thing." He pointed out that "by a mysterious decree of God" the plague was afflicting all peoples, including Jews; that it raged in places where no Jews lived, and that elsewhere they were victims like everyone else; therefore the charge that they caused it was "without plausibility." He urged the clergy to take Jews under their protection as he himself offered to do in Avignon, but his voice was hardly heard against local animus [hatred].

A Series of Organized Massacres

In Basle on January 9, 1349, the whole community of several hundred Jews was burned in a wooden house especially constructed for the purpose on an island in the Rhine, and a decree was passed that no Jew should be allowed to settle in Basle for 200 years. In Strasbourg the Town Council, which opposed persecution, was deposed by vote of the guilds and another was elected, prepared to comply with the popular will. In February 1349, before the plague had yet reached the city, the Jews of Strasbourg, numbering 2,000, were taken to the burial ground, where all except those who accepted conversion were burned at rows of stakes erected to receive them. . . .

In Freiburg, Augsburg, Nürnberg, Munich, Königsberg, Regensburg, and other centers, the Jews were slaughtered with a thoroughness that seemed to seek the final solution. At Worms in March 1349 the Jewish community of 400 . . . turned to an old tradition and burned themselves to death inside their own houses rather than be killed by their enemies. The larger community of Frankfurt-am-Main took the same way in July, setting fire to part of the city by their flames. . . . In Mainz, which had the largest Jewish community in Europe, its members turned at last to self-defense. With arms collected in advance they killed 200 of the mob, an act which only served to bring down upon them a furious onslaught by the townspeople in revenge for the death of Christians. The Jews fought until overpowered; then retreating to their homes, they too set their own fires. Six thousand were said to have perished at Mainz on August 24, 1349. Of 3,000 Jews at Erfurt, none was reported to have survived.

Completeness is rare in history, and Jewish chroniclers may have shared the medieval addiction to sweeping numbers. Usually a number saved themselves by conversion, and groups of refugees were given shelter by Rupert of the Palatinate and other princes. Duke Albert II of Austria, grand-uncle of Enguerrand VII, was one of the few who took measures effective enough to protect the Jews from assault in his territories. The last pogroms [organized massacres] took place in Antwerp and in Brussels where in December 1349 the entire Jewish community was exterminated. By the time the plague had passed, few Jews were left in Germany or the Low Countries. . . .

Homeless ghosts, the Jews filtered back from eastern Europe, where the expelled had gone. Two Jews reappeared in Erfurt as visitors in 1354 and, joined by others, started a resettlement three years later. By 1365 the community numbered 86 taxable hearths and an additional number of poor households below the tax-paying level. Here and elsewhere they returned to live in weakened and fearful communities on worse terms and in greater segregation than before. Well-poisoning and its massacres had fixed the malevolent image of the Jew into a stereotype. Because Jews were useful, towns which had enacted statutes of banishment invited or allowed their re-entry, but imposed new disabilities. Former contacts of scholars, physicians, and financial "court Jews" with the Gentile community faded. The period of the Jews' medieval flourishing was over. The walls of the ghetto, though not yet physical, had risen.

Chapter 2

The Economic and Cultural Impact of the Black Death

Turning|Points
IN WORLD HISTORY

The Black Death's Impact on Economics and Population

David Herlihy

This essay, one of the most important ever written about the Black Death, is by David Herlihy (who died in 1991), a former and highly distinguished professor of history at Brown University. He begins with a brief description of Europe's economic situation just prior to the onset of the Black Death. Then he discusses various economic changes caused by the loss of so many people to the disease in so short a time, supporting his arguments with excerpts from contemporary sources, including the *Decameron*, by the renowned fourteenth-century Italian writer Giovanni Boccaccio. For example, says Herlihy, there was an immediate demand for more people in certain professions such as gravedigging. And the huge labor losses resulting from the death toll made laborers rarer and therefore worth more, so the cost of labor rose sharply. Finally, Herlihy examines the epidemic's demographic impact, explaining natural population checks and how they affected various groups, especially the rich versus the poor.

Europe, before the Black Death assaulted it, was a very crowded continent. But despite the pressure on the land, stability prevailed. For fifty, perhaps one hundred years before 1348, the population had registered no significant gains. Food costs were high and famines frequent, but they did not send the population plummeting. The economy was saturated; nearly all available resources were committed to the effort of producing the food, clothing, and shelter needed to support the packed communities. Agriculture was mobilized

Reprinted by permission of the publisher from *The Black Death and the Transformation of the West*, by David Herlihy (Cambridge, MA: Harvard University Press). Copyright ©1997 by the President and Fellows of Harvard College. *Endnotes in the original have been omitted in this reprint.*

for the production of cereals, the basic foodstuff, and cultivation had extended to the limits of the workable land. Un-
doubtedly, vast numbers of Europeans lived in deep depriva-
tion. But despite misery and hunger, the pressure of human
numbers went unrelieved. The civilization that this economy supported, the civilization of the central Middle Ages,
might have maintained itself for the indefinite future. That
did not happen; an exogenous [outside, foreign] factor, the
Black Death, broke the . . . deadlock. And in doing so it gave
to Europeans the chance to rebuild their society along much
different lines.

The salient effects of the Black Death on the economic
and demographic systems of medieval Europe can be described with some certainty: the surviving evidence is reasonably abundant. Many contemporary witnesses commented on
human behavior at the workplace and marketplace in the
wake of epidemics. Even some quantitative data, chiefly price
citations, have survived. Several historians have used these
materials, and they are in considerable agreement as to the
nature and direction of economic change in the late Middle
Ages. The demographic system operating in medieval Europe is much harder to investigate. Records that could tell us
how medieval people married and reproduced are notori-
ously scarce and nearly always subject to diverse interpreta-
tions. Nonetheless, I shall argue here that the demographic
system of the Middle Ages, which I envisage as formed of the
relationships among deaths, marriages, and births, all subject
to the economic performance, was also profoundly altered in
this period of plague.

Short-Term Effects on Society

In considering the effect of the epidemics upon the economy, it is necessary to distinguish short-term and long-term
repercussions. The chief short-term repercussion was shock.
And shock in turn broke the continuities of economic life
and disrupted established routines of work and service. The
high mortalities left numerous posts in society unfilled and
services unperformed. According to Boccaccio, many con-
curred "that against plagues no medicine was better than or

even equal to simple flight." The retreat of the ten young Florentines to a country villa, portrayed in the *Decameron*, is a fictional but still typical example of this popular response to epidemic. The desertion of towns and cities, through death and flight, threatened communities with chaos.

How, under such conditions, could an organized economy be maintained? Many contemporaries affirm that it was not maintained, that workers either died or fled their posts, or simply refused to perform, preferring to indulge their appetites while they still had the chance. Peasants, according to Boccaccio, "just like the townspeople became lax in their ways and neglected their chores as if they expected death that very day.". . .

The epidemics also greatly enlarged the demand for certain types of services. The records mention most often the need for gravediggers, physicians, and priests.

Gravediggers gained a special prominence at a time when people died each day by the hundreds. The task of burying the dead apparently gave employment to marginal social groups, poor rustics, beggars, and the urban jobless. Boccaccio implies that gravediggers who worked for pay were unknown at Florence before the Black Death. He calls them "a species of vulture born from the lowly."

Physicians too were in demand. Boccaccio again laments that "the numbers [of physicians] had increased enormously because the ranks of the qualified were invaded by people, both men and women, who had never received any training in medicine." His allusion to women carers of the sick is especially noteworthy Another profession whose numbers proved inadequate for the services required was the clergy. Many priests had died, and many fled the contagion. Who would administer the Church's last rites to the many who were dying? . . .

The legal systems of late medieval Europe also had to respond to the extraordinary social situation created by an epidemic. Under conditions of plague, certain "privileges," as they were known in the legal language, went into effect. Women, for example, could now serve as witnesses, and scribes not formally admitted into the guild of notaries could draw up legal contracts. Society needed certain services, and at these moments of crisis it had to allow even the unlicensed or people believed to be incompetent to perform them.

More Young and Old People

Over the long term, the relaxation of the pressure of human numbers created serious problems for the economy. The chief problems were the drastic decrease in the number of workers, and the abbreviated span of years over which they remained productive. The plagues radically reduced the average duration of life. To the best of our knowledge, life expectancies in the good years of the thirteenth century were between 35 and 40 years. The ferocious epidemics of the late fourteenth century cut that figure to below 20; after 1400, as the population achieved a new equilibrium at very low levels, it extended to about 30 years. These figures necessarily affected the balances between young and old, and also between producers and dependents.

At Florence, a survey redacted in 1427 to 1430, called the Catasto, gives the ages of a large population of some 260,000 persons, in both cities and countryside. It thus allows us to see the demographic contours of a community that had within the lifetime of some of its members endured repeated epidemics, including the Black Death of 1348. The age pyramid of the Tuscan population is very distorted. Old persons age 60 or above are surprisingly numerous. They constitute nearly 15 percent of the community—a proportion one would expect to find in a modern Western population with a low birth rate. How did Tuscany accumulate such large numbers of the aged? The answer seems to be that those in the last stages of life were in part survivors of a time when the total community was much bigger than in 1427. It also suggests that the plague preyed on the young rather than the mature. If a person survived one major epidemic, the chances improved that he or she would survive the next.

The number of children and youths up to age 19 was also very large, forming about 44 percent of the population—again a figure surprising for its size. So large a proportion of

the young is normally found in a rapidly growing community, but Tuscany in 1427 was still barely maintaining its
numbers. The adult and productive members of society,
those between 20 and 59, were thus a minority of about 41
percent. . . . Adults in their productive years thus bore a huge
burden of dependents. Moreover, the wealth and effort invested in the rearing of children remained in significant
measure wasted. Death ruthlessly thinned the ranks of the
young before they could repay to society the resources and
energy devoted to them. . . .

Higher Prices and Living Standards

But, over the long run . . . [depopulation] conferred advan-
tages too. Above all it freed resources. The collapse of population liberated land for uses other than the cultivation of
grains. It could be turned to pasturage or to forests. In the
past mills and mill sites had served predominantly for the
grinding of grain. They now could be enlisted for other uses:
the fulling of cloth, the operation of bellows, the sawing of
wood. Even as the population shrank, the possibility of developing a more diversified economy was enhanced.

Price movements provide our best evidence of the direc-
tions of long-term economic trends in the late Middle Ages.
The immediate effect of the Black Death upon prices was to
produce general inflation. The Florentine Matteo Villani,
writing in 1363, presents an apt analysis of price movements
since 1348:

> . . . It was thought that there ought to be wealth and abun-
> dance of clothing, and of all the other things that the human
> body needs . . . but the opposite happened. . . . Most things
> cost two times or more what they cost before the epidemic.
> And labor, and the manufactures of every art and profession
> increased in disorderly fashion to double the price.

This general inflation persisted until the last decades of
the fourteenth century, and indicates that under the shock of
plague production in town and countryside had fallen even
more rapidly than the population.

Of all commodity prices, the most important, indeed the

usual reference base for all others, was that of wheat. Wheat prices were everywhere high in Europe before the Black Death, reflecting the huge numbers of consumers and the intensive cultivation of grain, even on marginal soils. Wheat prices also increased after the Black Death. In England, Normandy, the Ile-de-France, Alsace, Flanders, and Spain, they remained high until about 1375. In Tuscany the period of inflation persisted even longer, to about 1395. . . .

The price of animal products—meat, sausage, cheese and the like—also remained relatively high. Europeans, even as their numbers declined, were living better. Many moralists complain of the extravagant tastes for food and attire which the lower social orders now manifested. [Italian commentator] Matteo Villani remarks: "The common people, by reason of the abundance and superfluity that they found, would no longer work at their accustomed trades; they wanted the dearest and most delicate foods . . . while children and common women clad themselves in all the fair and costly garments of the illustrious who had died." Conspicuous consumption by the humble threatened to erase the visible marks of social distinctions and to undermine the social order. The response of the alleged prodigality in food and clothing was sumptuary laws, which governments enacted all over Europe in the fourteenth and fifteenth centuries. They tried to regulate fashions, such as the size of sleeves or the length of trains in women's dresses; meals, such as the food to be served at weddings; or customs, such as the number of mourners who could attend a funeral. The repetition of these laws suggests their futility. High wages to the poor and improved living standards came to be irremediable facts of late medieval economic and social life.

The price of wool moved erratically, but was strong enough to stimulate a widespread conversion from plowland to meadow. Moreover, one or two shepherds could guard hundreds of sheep, and this extensive use of the land saved the costs of hiring expensive tillers. Manufactured products also held their value better than wheat. But in the late Middle Ages, silk challenged wool as the most active branch of the textile production, again indicating smaller, but richer markets.

Cheap Land and Capital, Better Technology

Besides commodity prices, the costs of the classical "factors of production"—labor, land, and capital—also responded to the new conditions. Of these production costs, the one most dramatically affected was that of labor. The falling numbers of renters and workers increased the strength of their negotiating position in bargaining with landlords and entrepreneurs. Agricultural rents collapsed after the Black Death, and wages in the towns soared, to two and even three times the levels they had held in the crowded thirteenth century. . . .

Governments tried to cap the swell in wages and to shore up the shrinking rents. They sought to hold prices and wages to previous levels and insisted that workers accept any employment offered them. But they succeeded only in sowing discontent and in provoking social uprisings in city and countryside. The value of land diminished. We do not know a great deal of the costs of capital. But references in chronicles such as Matteo Villani's to the accumulation of inheritances suggest that capital too became cheaper in the contracting community.

The different movements of factor costs favored a policy of factor substitution. In particular, cheap land and capital were widely substituted for expensive labor. In effect, the conversion of land from wheat fields into pasturage is an example of factor substitution, and many others could be cited. In agriculture, the purchase of oxen to aid the peasant in plowing and to increase his supply of fertilizer enabled him to work more productively. According to Matteo Villani, Tuscan peasants would not accept a lease unless the landlord provided oxen and seed—in other words, increased capital. In the urban economy, the substitution of capital for labor meant the purchase of better tools or machines—devices that enabled the artisan to work more efficiently. Frequently too, the policy of factor substitution involved technological innovation, the development of entirely new tools and machines. High labor costs promised big rewards to the inventors of labor-saving devices. Chiefly for this reason, the late Middle Ages were a period of impressive technological achievement.

New methods of reproducing the written word offer a clear instance of capital replacing labor by virtue of technology. The growth of universities in the twelfth and thirteenth centuries and the expanding numbers of literate laymen generated a strong demand for books. Numerous scribes were employed to copy manuscripts. At Paris, for example, in the thirteenth century, manuscripts were divided into quires and given to separate scribes, who assiduously reproduced them. The parts were then combined into the finished book. As long as wages were low, this method of reproduction based on intensive human labor was satisfactory enough.

But the late medieval population plunge raised labor costs, and also raised the premium to be claimed by the one who could devise a cheaper way of reproducing books. Johann Gutenberg's invention of printing on the basis of movable metal type in 1453 was only the culmination of many experiments carried on across the previous century. . . . He and all the early printers were businessmen. Printing shops required considerable capital to set up their presses and to market their books. But they were able to multiply texts with unprecedented accuracy and speed, and at greatly reduced costs. The advent of printing is thus a salient example of the policy of factor substitution which was transforming the late medieval economy. . . .

A more diversified economy, a more intensive use of capital, a more powerful technology, and a higher standard of living for the people—these seem the salient characteristics of the late medieval economy, after it recovered from the plague's initial shock and learned to cope with the problems raised by diminished numbers. Specific changes in technology are of course primarily attributable to the inventive genius of individuals. But the huge losses caused by plague and the high cost of labor were the challenge to which these efforts responded. Plague, in sum, broke the . . . [population] deadlock of the thirteenth century, which threatened to hold Europe in its traditional ways for the indefinite future. The Black Death devastated society, but it did not cripple human resilience.

Natural Checks on Population Growth

Another set of institutions and practices reformed in the wake of the epidemics was the demographic system. To examine the changes in the European demographic system across the

late Middle Ages requires first that we understand the principles that govern demographic systems of any sort. People are
born and people die, and these events affect the size of the
community. But the size of the community also affects these
events, through a kind of feedback mechanism, in the language of contemporary systems analysis. Many observers in
both the ancient world and the Middle Ages recognized, for
example, that the earth could not support infinite human
numbers; when overburdened, it periodically purged itself of
excess, through famines, wars, plagues, floods, earthquakes,
and other natural disasters.

It remained, however, for [eighteenth-century British
economist] Thomas Malthus to interpret the relation of community size to vital events in terms of an overarching system.
Populations, he argued, inevitably grow faster than their supplies of food, the former tending to increase geometrically,
the latter only arithmetically. Predictably, the population
would at some point surpass the numbers that its resources
could adequately feed. It would then face a reckoning. The
reckoning took the form of famines, malnutrition, plagues,
and wars, which raised the death rate to a level higher than
the birth rate, and thus cut down the size of the community.
Malthus called the mechanisms by which growth was re-
strained and reversed "checks.". . .

Malthus also recognized another type of check that controlled human numbers. These he called "preventive
checks." The cost of food, rising as population increased, reduced real wages, as workers had to devote ever greater
shares of their disposable income to subsistence. But in some
cultures, declining real wages also inhibited marriages, as
only those young couples with the means of supporting a
family could allow themselves to marry and to set up a new
household. In preventing or delaying marriages, this sort of
check lowered the birth rate as well. It thus was capable of
controlling growth and of keeping the population well
within the size its resources could comfortably support. The
community need not test the ceiling of subsistence. . . .

It is certain that some forms of preventive checks func-
tioned even in the Middle Ages. The chief evidence for this

comes from the consistent association in medieval household surveys of wealth and household size. The earliest large survey of a medieval community we possess is the *polyptych* of the abbot Irminon, who presided over the monastery of St. Germain de Près near Paris in the early ninth century. The *polyptych* includes nearly 2,000 entries describing the monastery's possessions in the neighborhood of Paris, some 1,647 of which inventory dependent farms, specify their size, and take note of the serfs and their families who worked and lived on the farms. There are many difficulties with these data, and the survey does not support refined analysis. But if we crudely compare the size of the plowlands, vineyards, and meadows with the number of persons settled upon them, an unmistakable association emerges. Those households with five or fewer units of land show an average size of 3.9 persons; those with six to ten units, 5.43 members; those with 11 to 15, 7.04 members; those with 16 to 20, 8.83; and those with more than 20, 10.07. The progression is clear: the more land, the larger the household living from it.

This close association of extent of land with size of household, evident in our earliest surveys, is very nearly a general rule of household organization in the Middle Ages. It means that the possession of a big farm made possible the support of a big family, but the converse also holds true: those with little land could afford to maintain only small households. . . .

Rich Versus Poor

Medieval observers shared the view that the poor were much more susceptible than the rich to the ravages of famine and plague. At Florence, Matteo Villani claims that the Black Death of 1348 wiped out the poor completely—those who two decades before were more than 17,000. "And the mendicant poor were almost all dead," he states. "And there were not at that time," he elsewhere observes, any "needy poor."

The presumption that the poor were the chosen victims of hunger and disease persists into early modern times. In the seventeenth century, a Florentine doctor named Alessandro Righi compared the body physical with the body social. The human body was composed of both noble and ignoble parts. The noble parts were the heart, the brain, the liver, and the principal organs. They had the power to expel poisonous substances to the periphery. The ignoble parts, the glands and the skin, had no such powers and thus became the receptacles of the poisons dispatched from the center. So it was with the city. The nobles were the principal organs, and the poor the ignoble skin and glands. "Nor can they," writes the doctor, "transmit [the poison] to others, and therefore it is necessary, that if anything evil is in the city, they receive it and hold it as they are the glands of the city."

The demographic system prevailing in medieval society appears to have been two-tiered. At the bottom of the social ladder, positive checks primarily controlled the numbers of the impoverished. Above this social sector were the middle classes and the wealthy, among whom preventive checks had become the more effective means of regulating numbers. In the Catasto of the city of Florence, dated 1427, wealth shows its characteristic correlation with household size, but, significantly, its influence becomes evident only above a threshold of approximately 400 florins in assessed household wealth. Somewhere between 30 and 40 percent of the households fell below the threshold when wealth began to have a visible influence on household organization and demographic behavior. The demographic system operating in Florence in 1427 still looks to be two-tiered, but now most households had passed under the control of preventive, not positive, checks.

The great population debacle of the late Middle Ages did not, in sum, introduce an entirely new demographic system. But it did redistribute the population between the two tiers of the traditional system. Depopulation gave access to farms and remunerative jobs to a larger percentage of the population. High wages and low rents also raised the standard of living for substantial numbers. They became acquainted with a style of life that they or their children would not want easily to abandon. For a significantly larger part of society, the care of property and the defense of living standards were tightly joined with decisions to marry and to reproduce. . . . Out of the havoc of plague, Europe adopted what can well be called the modern Western mode of demographic behavior.

Educational, Agricultural, and Architectural Impact of the Black Death

Philip Ziegler

In this excerpt from his widely read and respected 1969 book on the Black Death, British scholar Philip Ziegler examines how the disaster affected various aspects of education. Many scholars died in the epidemic, he points out, and numerous new universities were established in its wake. But the biggest change was a rise in the teaching and stature of national languages, such as English, German, and Italian, as opposed to Latin, which was more of an *inter*national language. Also, says Ziegler, the great plague brought about a significant redistribution of many of the lands that were formerly connected to large manorial estates. By contrast, Ziegler contends that the Black Death had much less impact on changing architectural styles than many scholars had previously suggested. He argues, for instance, that the transition from the English Decorated style (early to mid-1300s), an ornate form of Gothic architecture, to the Perpendicular style (late 1300s to early 1700s), a Gothic phase stressing vertical lines, was only partially influenced by the Black Death.

Such modifications of the social structure of the country were bound to find their reflection in almost every sphere of human activity. There can have been very little in English life which survived the Black Death wholly unchanged, though in some fields the changes were at first almost imperceptible and only gradually revealed their true significance.

The Rise of National Languages

The world of education, through its dependence on a comparatively small group of learned men of whom the most powerful and distinguished were often also among the oldest, was peculiarly sensitive to the impact of the plague. Mortality among men of learning had been calamitously high. Four of Europe's thirty universities vanished in the middle of the fourteenth century: no one can be sure that the Black Death was responsible but it would be over-cautious to deny that it must have played a part. Arezzo ceased to exist a few years later; Siena closed for several years. The chancellor of Oxford petitioned the King 'showing that the university is ruined and enfeebled by the pestilence and other causes, so that its estate can hardly be maintained or protected.' The students of Avignon addressed the Pope: '. . . at a time when the university body of your studium . . . is deprived of all lectures, since the whole number has been left desolate by the death from pestilence of doctors, licentiates, bachelors and students. . . .'

Into this vacuum there was ample scope for new ideas and doctrines to infiltrate. In England one important by-product, caused in part at least by the shortage of people qualified to teach in French after the Black Death, was the growth of education in the vernacular [common language of a country] and of translation from Latin direct to English. . . .

It would, of course, be absurd to attribute to any individual or to the Black Death itself the full responsibility for a change which had already started even before 1348 and, in the end, would inevitably have carried all before it. But it would also be a mistake to discount unduly the importance of the Black Death in removing so many of those who would have been a barrier to reform and in making it, in purely practical terms, far more difficult to carry on along the old path. . . .

The growth of a literature in the vernacular was bound, in the end, to mean the disappearance of Latin as a medium of communication. It took an unconscionably long time a-dying; vestigial relics are, indeed, still said to linger on in England to-day in certain of the more antique seats of learning. But its monopoly was broken. English arose; the symbol of a new nationalism, to take its place in the law courts as the instrument for the transaction of business and for the conduct of relationships even in the most polite society. It was nationalism that dictated the use of English rather than the use of English which created nationalism, but the two fostered each other and grew side by side. Neither the growth of a national language nor of a national spirit can be said to be a uniquely English phenomenon. The sort of generalisa-

Changing English Architectural Styles

The late and distinguished architectural historian Nikolaus Pevsner here supports Ziegler's contention that changing English architectural styles were only marginally influenced by the Black Death. When did the one phase end and the other begin? . . . British architectural style shortly after [the erection of] Bristol [Cathedral in the early 1300s] and Ely [Cathedral, ca. 1321–1349] changed once more and changed most signally. The change is so obvious that, while for the Continent [i.e., the European mainland] the terms High and Late Gothic are sufficient to indicate the chief stages, in England tradition has for more than a hundred years preferred a division into three Gothic phases: Early English, Decorated, and Perpendicular. Early English was at an end when the Angel Choir was growing. Decorated is the style of Bristol and Ely. Perpendicular corresponds to what we have seen of Late Gothic in Germany and Spain, and it is a contribution of equal national vigour. Once it had been created by a few strong-minded, clear-headed architects, it brushed aside all the vagaries of Decorated and settled down to a long, none too adventurous development of plain-spoken idiom, sober and wide-awake. People have tried to connect the coming of this new style with the Black Death of 1349. This is wrong; for it is there in all its perfection as early as 1331–7 in the south transept and as early as 1337–77 in the choir of Gloucester Cathedral.

Nikolaus Pevsner, *An Outline of European Architecture.* Baltimore: Penguin Books, 1943, p. 150.

tion with which we are dealing here could be applied . . . to what we now mean by France, Italy or Germany. But nowhere else was the evolution so pronounced or the relevance of the Black Death so clearly marked.

'We must not think,' wrote Dr Pantin [W.A. Pantin, *The English Church and the Continent: The Later Middle Ages*], 'that "nationalism" was something invented at the Renaissance or even in the later middle ages . . . since the eleventh century there had been highly organized "national" states and deep political and racial divisions and rivalries and antipathies. . . .' One must not give the Black Death too much prominence in an evolution which has edged forward fitfully over many centuries, yet it would be quite as foolish to ignore its role and it is surely permissible, too, to see its by-products in the field of learning as one of the more decisive catalytic factors. In England too, it was more immediately apparent that the weakening of the international language was a blow to the universal Church. It would be a grotesque over-statement to claim that, if the English had continued to speak French and write Latin, there would have been no Reformation, but, like most over-statements, it would contain some elements of truth.

New Universities

In the long run the English Universities had no cause to regret the temporary havoc which the plague caused in their workings. The shortage of clergy and lay clerks was so conspicuous that the provision of replacements became an urgent need. At Cambridge the reaction was swift. Trinity Hall, Gonville Hall and Corpus Christi were all founded as a consequence, Corpus Christi, at least, as a direct consequence of the Black Death. In the deed of 6 February, 1350, by which Bishop Bateman established Trinity Hall it was specifically laid down that the purpose of the new college was to make good the appalling losses which the clergy in England and, in particular, East Anglia had suffered. The motives for founding Corpus Christi were slightly less altruistic. The members of the trade guilds found that, with the shortage of clergy after the plague, it cost them too much to have masses said for their departed members. By establishing a college they calculated that they would acquire a plentiful supply of cheap labour among the students. So deep a scar did the plague leave that even in 1441, at the foundation of King's, the statutes, though in general terms, reiterated a reference to the need to repair the ravages of a century before.

Oxford was somewhat slower off the mark. It took ten years and a second attack of the plague to induce Simon Islip, Archbishop of Canterbury, to follow Bishop Bateman's lead. '. . . I, Simon . . . in view of the fact that in particular those who are truly learned and accomplished in every kind of learning have been largely exterminated in the epidemics, and that, because of the lack of opportunity, very few are coming forward at present to carry on such studies . . .' heartily support a gift of money made to my 'new college of Canterbury at Oxford.'

Similarly, a few years later, William of Wykeham, wishing to cure 'the general disease of the clerical army, which we have observed to be grievously wounded owing to the small number of the clergy, as a result of pestilences, wars and other miseries of the world' founded New College to repair the deficiency. But New College owed more to the Black Death than the inspiration for its creation. According to tradition . . . New College garden was the site of Oxford's largest plague pit, an area formerly covered by houses but depopulated by the epidemic and converted to its grisly purpose. The ill wind also blew good to Merton College since the sharp drop in population allowed it to buy, at a bargain price, almost all the land between the City Wall and St Frideswides; an investment whose increasing value must have done much to solace future generations for the tribulations of their ancestors.

Land Redistribution

It would have been extraordinary if the striking changes which the Black Death had helped to evolve in the relationship between landlord and tenant had not produced perceptible results in the practice of agriculture and even the appearance of the English countryside. The crucial consequence of the epidemic was that much land fell free and that the lord not only did not wish to farm it himself but was often anxious to divest himself even of that part of the land which had formed part of his demesne [estate] before 1348. The tenements of those who died and left no heir were therefore available for distribution among those who remained. Sometimes such tenements might be taken up by immigrants who had sickened of their own, less fertile holdings and let the wilderness take over its own again. But more often the lands of the deceased were carved up among the surviving tenants of the village.

Each tenant, therefore, was likely to have a larger holding than before and, in the fluid conditions which prevailed after the plague, these could be organised into more coherent and viable blocks than had been possible under the old pattern of cultivation. The tendency was reinforced where the landlord alienated his demesne. Once a tenant was established in possession of a coherent parcel of land, then it was inevitable that he would seek to demarcate it more clearly and organise his different activities on a more workable basis. It would be wrong to speak of any dramatic and sudden switch; it took generations to transform the face of the countryside. But the hedged fields of England can plausibly be argued to have had their genesis in the aftermath of the Black Death and though such changes would, in the long run, have been inevitable, their evolution might otherwise have followed a distinct and far more protracted path. . . .

Architectural Impact Exaggerated?

A field in which the significance of the Black Death seems more significant in legend than in reality is that of architecture. The skilled masons capable of executing the fine traceries and, still more, the figure sculpture of the Decorated period were, it is contended, almost wiped out by the plague. Those who were left were too much in demand, too pressed for time, to be able to use their talents to the full. The new generation of masons, artisans rather than artists, were affected by the new mobility of labour which was so marked a feature of the post-plague period. Forced to work in a variety of stones, most of them unfamiliar, it was inevitable that the workmen should opt for less complicated and ambitious techniques. The result was a sharp fall in standards. . . .

There is, of course, something in this argument. Without doubt many skilled craftsmen died during the plague and were never replaced. With them died one of the glories of English religious architecture. There can be no absolute standard of beauty but most people would probably agree that York Minster would be more perfect a building if work had begun ten or twenty years before it did. As it was, work came to a sudden stop on the almost completed west front and nave. The choir had not yet been begun and no further progress was made till 1361. For its construction the old plans were scrapped and the Decorated style replaced by the formal stiffness of the Perpendicular. One reason at least for this must have been the technical impossibility of continuing to build a Decorated church when so many of the more experienced masons were dead.

But can a trend which led directly to the towers of Worcester, the west front of Beverley Minster or the nave of Canterbury, possibly be cited as evidence of inferior artistry? To suggest that the Perpendicular style was no more than a degenerate variant on the traditional Decorated would show a derisory misunderstanding of one of the noblest schools of English architecture. Nor should the significance of the Black Death be over-stated in an artistic revolution which had started twenty years before and which the calamities of the mid-fourteenth century checked but could not extinguish. The transept and choir of Gloucester, the cradle of Perpendicular, were completed in 1332 and, though the Black Death introduced economic and social factors which diffused the new fashion more widely, it would be misleading to suggest that those were of prime importance. 'Perpendicular,' wrote Mr Harvey [J. Harvey, *Gothic England*], 'was not the outcome of poverty and failure, but of riches and success. Only to a comparatively slight extent was its course changed by the coming of the Black Death, which did but accelerate a movement already in being.'

How the Black Death Affected the Church

Frederick F. Cartwright and Michael D. Biddiss

The Christian Church underwent material losses, including the death of many priests, nuns, and deacons, during the great fourteenth-century epidemic. It also suffered a severe loss of prestige, since the popular perception was that priests had been unable to intercede with God to stop the plague. In this excerpt from their book, *Disease in History*, noted medical historian Frederick F. Cartwright and Cambridge University history professor Michael D. Biddiss discuss these material losses and go on to suggest that resultant changes in religious thinking eventually contributed to the Reformation and emergence of Protestantism. Finally, Cartwright and Biddiss point out that one way the Church attempted to maintain its authority in the post-plague years was to continue to stifle creative thinking and learning. With minor exceptions, this discouraged needed advances in medical science for the next few centuries.

The Christian Church had risen to be a dominant power partly as a result of the earlier pestilences. It would be strange if so great a catastrophe as the Black Death did not exert some influence upon the authority of a religion which had now been established for 1,000 years. The remarkable grasp of the Church upon Europe enabled Christianity to weather the storm, but the authority of the Church did not survive the Black Death unscathed.

Up to a point, Church influence had been for the public good; she preserved a limited peace in times of strife, tried to impose a code of human behaviour, and acted as school-

Excerpted from *Disease and History*, by Frederick F. Cartwright, in collaboration with Michael D. Biddiss (New York: Dorset Press, 1972). Copyright ©1972 by Frederick F. Cartwright. Reprinted by permission of Frederick F. Cartwright.

mistress. The Church harnessed and nourished intellect, taught and provided administrators, lawyers and physicians, encouraged and preserved architecture, literature and art. But, although creative work might be encouraged, creative thought was more often sternly repressed. The doctrine of persecution formed an integral part of mediaeval Christianity and those whose written or spoken thoughts did not follow the rigid line permitted by the Church stood in danger of persecution as heretics.

Material Losses

In material matters the Church suffered badly from the Black Death. A great loss of manpower and impoverishment through inability to cultivate her vast tracts of land rendered her a less dominant power in 1350 than in 1346. But greater harm resulted from her helplessness in this time of disaster, a large loss of priests and monks, and her failure to control their successors. Parish priests, the best-loved of church workers, died by the hundreds and according to [contemporary English poet] William Langland their benefices were all too often hurriedly filled by 'numbers of youths, that had only devoted themselves for clerks by being shaven'. If Langland is to be believed—and there is no reason to disbelieve him—the friars, who had previously been renowned for holiness and charity, gave themselves up to 'gayness and gluttony', while country parsons and parish priests spent their time in London, touting for high places, instead of ministering to their parishioners. Langland specifically states in both instances that these abuses had multiplied 'sithen the pestilence time'.

Further, the very fact that the Church possessed the seeming advantage of being international or supra-national implied a threat to her power. In many countries, Germany and England for example, People and Church had been falling out of sympathy for a number of years. The national branches of the Church cried out for reform, but they had no power to reform themselves because they lacked autonomy; they were, in fact, outlying parts of a foreign organization of immense power and prestige.

Religious Deviations

For all these reasons, open opposition to the Church developed in the years immediately following the Black Death. Popular reaction can be measured by contrasting the murders of two prominent English churchmen. In 1170 the Archbishop of Canterbury was done to death as the result of some hasty words spoken by King Henry II; although Thomas à Becket's policy was not generally approved, public horror at this sacrilege forced the king to submit himself to humiliating penance. In 1381 a band of rebels seized the mild Simon Sudbury, Archbishop of Canterbury, and struck off his head on Tower Hill in London amid the ferocious applause of a great crowd. 'The relation of Church and people had undergone a profound change since the ancestors of these same men had knelt beside their ploughs to pray for the Holy Martyr, Thomas à Becket,' wrote [noted historian] G.M. Trevelyan.

The change was more profound than is suggested by the murder of Sudbury, Langland's disapproval or the deviant behaviour of flagellants. John Wyclif, born about 1320 and dying in 1384, was a notable theologian and Master of Balliol College, Oxford. He questioned Holy Church's hitherto unchallenged power. As well as demanding a vernacular [national language, rather than Latin] Order of Service and translating the Bible into English, he attacked the worship of images and relics, the sale of pardons and masses for the dead. Wyclif gained an immense following who became known as the Lollards. They were drawn not only from the common people, but from the nobility, the friars and some of the lesser clergy who had reason to dislike wealthy monks and bishops.

Wyclif was before his time. As the Church re-established its shaken authority, the Lollards became subject to persecution and were driven underground, to reappear in the reigns of Henry VII and VIII. Persecuted again, they re-emerged to combine with the Protestants of Martin Luther. Luther owed something to the teaching of the earlier reformer John Huss of Bohemia, and Huss, in turn, acknowledged himself a pupil of Wyclif. Thus it is not too much to claim that the

Protestant Reformation, the sailing of the Brownist Pilgrim Fathers in the *Mayflower* from Plymouth on 6 September 1620 and the foundation of Pennsylvania by the Quaker William Penn in 1681, can all be linked with the deviation from established religion that followed the disaster of the Black Death.

A Stranglehold on Medicine

One would have thought that so great a pestilence, in which physicians and priests alike proved useless, must have profoundly affected the development of the theocratic medical art. This is not so. Almost the only medical advance directly attributable to the Black Death is in the field of public health. In 1374 the Venetian republic appointed three officials whose duty was to inspect and to exclude all infected vessels from the ports. In 1377 Ragusa detained travellers from infected places for thirty days (*trentini giorni*). When this proved ineffective, the period of detention was lengthened to forty days (*quaranti giorni*); from this early preventive measure comes our modern word 'quarantine'.

Besides this, the Black Death added yet another saint to the Calendar. St Roch is the special patron of bubonic plague. A native of Montpellier, he nursed the sick during the Black Death in north Italy and himself fell a victim. Left to die, Roch was succoured by a dog and recovered. He returned to his home town but was suspected of being a spy and cast into prison, where he died. Here again is the pattern of mortal hurt, miraculous recovery, and ultimate death.

We should honour the Church for her unremitting care of the sick, but acknowledge that her influence upon medical and scientific advance was almost wholly evil. The 1,000-year repression of many forms of creative thought between the fall of Rome and the Renaissance provides a miserable picture of sterile plagiarism [copying earlier ideas and writings rather than initiating original ones]. Great schools of medicine were founded—Salerno and Bologna in Italy, Paris and Montpellier in France—but the teaching in those schools was an uncritical reiteration of ancient theories, and research took the form of disputations upon the exact meaning of a text. The vast medical literature of this long period contains many original observations but scarcely any original thought; it is little better than a series of compilations, the substance derived from Latin texts of first-century authors and their Islamic commentators. There are, of course, occasional flashes of the divine fire, for no weight of repression will ever stifle criticism entirely. Thus Mundinus of Bologna defied the ban upon human dissection and did something to restore the science of anatomy to the standard reached by Greek workers about 300 B.C. Another flame in the darkness is Roger Bacon of Oxford and Paris, a philosopher rather than a physician and certainly an original thinker, but his originality earned him imprisonment for the last thirteen years of his life.

The habit of thought engendered by theocratic intolerance stifled medical advance until the end of the fifteenth century. [The ancient Greek physician] Galen remained the unquestioned authority. This dominance of one man would have been bad enough in itself, but the texts of Galen had been so debased as to be almost worthless. The true teachings of Galen were not restored until too late when, at the end of the fifteenth century, a new way of thinking opened up great vistas of learning and beauty. The wonderful phenomenon of the Renaissance was not merely a revival of classical culture; it was a change in the whole outlook of thinking men, who demanded escape from the tyranny of dogmatism, from the limitations of thought imposed by the Church. Although the ghost of Galen was not laid until William Harvey disproved his doctrine of the ebb-and-flow movement of blood in the seventeenth century, it was the Renaissance that finally broke the Church's stranglehold upon medicine.

The Plague and Other Killer Diseases in Modern Times

Turning Points
IN WORLD HISTORY

The New Epidemic

Arno Karlen

As noted scholar and educator Arno Karlen explains in this dramatic and eye-opening essay, humanity's battle against highly infectious and destructive diseases like the Black Death is far from over. Karlen expertly chronicles the demise of the unbridled medical optimism of the nineteenth and early twentieth centuries, an era in which it appeared that science was on the verge of eradicating most diseases. In fact, humanity is presently under attack by a barrage of diseases, some old and many new, including AIDS, herpes and other sexually transmitted pathogens, and exotic and deadly fevers and influenza. In a thought-provoking conclusion, Karlen places much of the blame for the new epidemic crisis on the rapid global environmental changes caused by modern human civilization. Diseases are "a natural, in fact necessary part of life," he states. "New ones are always coming into existence, [and] most change with time." Thus, despite the huge strides made by modern science, the potential exists for new mass onslaughts of pestilence, one or more of which might someday rival the Black Death's terrible fourteenth-century visitation.

An alarming tide of new and resurgent diseases has been rising around the world for decades. Now it advances faster than ever. This signals a crisis in the history of the human species. We have brought it on by rending the fabric of our environment, changing our behavior, and ironically, by our inventiveness in increasing the length and quality of our lives.

Until quite recently, few people seemed aware of this epidemic of epidemics. Even among doctors and researchers, concern was rare. Almost twenty years ago, I told friends

---

Reprinted from chapter 1 of *Man and Microbes*, by Arno Karlen (New York: Putnam, 1995). Copyright ©1995 by Quantum Research Associates, Inc. Used by permission of Jonathan Dolger Literary Agency on behalf of the author.

that I was thinking of writing about why so many new diseases were appearing. Most of my friends were puzzled. A few asked if I meant Legionnaires' disease and Lyme disease, both of which had lately appeared. I said yes, those and many others. I began gathering material.

Five years later, I wanted to write a book about the emergence of slow viruses, and the major epidemics I felt sure would follow. AIDS had not yet been identified and named. No publisher was interested. I was told that this could interest only specialists.

In 1990, I outlined this book. Its central idea still puzzled many people. When I said it was about new diseases and where they come from, most said, "You mean AIDS." A few, with more than average interest in such things, mentioned Lassa, Ebola, and Marburg fevers. Yes, I said, and many, many more.

When I began work on the book, I predicted to its publisher that before it appeared, at least two or three new epidemic diseases would make headlines; so would several old ones once thought defeated but now out of control again. Since then, a lethal hantavirus has appeared in the Four Corners region of the American Southwest. A new strain of *Escherichia coli* bacteria has caused widespread illness and death, raising worries about the safety of the nation's food supply. There have been upsurges in cases of measles, drug-resistant tuberculosis, diphtheria, and cholera. The appearance of a new, highly virulent strain of cholera bacilli may have marked the start of another global epidemic. And pneumonic plague broke out for the first time in a hundred years, in India.

For each new disease known to the general public, there are a dozen others; the wheels of biological change keep turning faster. The shared evolution of humans and microbes has accelerated to a frenzied pace, because of changes we have made in our environment and our lifestyles. Much has been written about AIDS, but far less about other new diseases. The scientific and historical research is fragmented, like pieces of a mosaic rarely assembled in more than bits and patches. In the past few years, a handful of books for nonspecialists have appeared, about one disease or another, about emerging viruses and the increase of microbial resistance to drugs. But without seeing the larger evolutionary picture, we cannot respond wisely to these challenges to our health and survival. The cost in suffering and deaths will be devastating.

The Fourth Horseman of Doom

We have been slow to understand that we live in a new bio-cultural era. For decades we cherished the myth that infectious diseases were fading forever. This was a posture born of inherited optimism. The nineteenth century generated an almost religious faith in social, scientific, and technological progress. Such optimism enabled people to call the slaughter of 1914–1918 a war to end all wars The two great global epidemics of that era, typhus and type A influenza, each killed 20 million people or more, dwarfing the toll of combat, without blunting popular faith in medical progress.

At first, events seemed to justify such optimism. More than a half-century would pass before the arrival of AIDS, another epidemic that kills by the millions. Those decades brought cleaner food and water, better living conditions, polio vaccine, antibiotics, the eradication of smallpox, and huge reductions of such killers as tuberculosis, cholera, and syphilis. Agricultural abundance soared in the developed world, and then in developing nations. The deaths of infants and small children, for so long routine events, became unusual tragedies. Life spans increased, and in some places almost doubled. World War II was the first major war in which epidemics took far fewer casualties than battle.

Now, just a few generations later, it is difficult to appreciate how astonishing all this was. For 10,000 years, since the first hunter-gatherers settled in villages, infections had killed more people than war and famine. Suddenly, by the 1930s, a new era of fitness and longevity was arriving; to many, it promised an end to all infectious disease. Pestilence, the Fourth Horseman of the Apocalypse, which a generation earlier had galloped the world, seemed a quaint bogey. Cities of the future were portrayed sparkling under plastic bubbles no germ or poison could penetrate. From now on, medicine's great task would be treating cancer, clogged arteries, stress, and the other so-called diseases of civilization and of aging. When fluoridation [the sterilization of water supplies] arrived, after World War II, it seemed that we would even reach vigorous old age with our teeth intact.

In 1969, the U.S. surgeon general, Dr. William H. Stewart, told the nation that it had already seen most of the frontiers in the field of contagious disease. Epidemiology [the study of the causes and controls of diseases] seemed destined to become a scientific backwater. A decade later, the governments of the United States, Canada, and Great Britain announced that their citizens must recognize a radical transformation; they were threatened no longer by microbes but by their own heedlessness. Drinking, smoking, and driving without seat belts had replaced bubonic plague, smallpox, and cholera. The authorities had a point, but they failed to mention such expanding avenues of infection as drugs, sex, rapid world travel, new medical procedures, and environmental degradation.

The Dream of a Sanitary Utopia Shattered

In fact, as developed nations indulged visions of an antiseptic age, new diseases were already appearing. At first they arose mostly in remote parts of Africa and Asia. Some took small tolls; others caught the eyes of only the dwindling ranks of specialists in tropical medicine and epidemiology. In the 1960s and 1970s, new diseases struck with greater impact and visibility. Old ones reappeared as vicious changelings, resistant to drugs that had once controlled them. Syphilis, malaria, and measles made frightening comebacks. Even bubonic plague popped up sporadically in Sun Belt suburbs, and among American troops serving in Vietnam.

A few scientists voiced urgent worry, but they went largely unheeded. Most of their colleagues, like most of the public, still thought the world was advancing into a golden biomedical era. Some predicted healthy life spans in triple digits. In retrospect, such confidence seems not only foolhardy but arrogant.

The 1980s brought more reports of new diseases, drug-resistant bacteria, and thriving disease carriers, from mosquitoes to household pets. Infections once limited to small areas were spreading; Lyme disease and Rocky Mountain spotted fever, once local concerns, ranged from coast to coast. AIDS became, inevitably, a national obsession. At the same time, a trickle of environmental warnings swelled to a dire stream. Pollutants, carcinogens, and ecological insults from the groundwater to the ozone layer were said to threaten the health of the entire biosphere. Yet few people made the connection between environmental and epidemiological changes

In the 1990s, we can see that for each disease conquered, another has emerged or reemerged. Scores of infections have shattered the dream of a sanitary utopia, where only genetic controls on aging limit the human life span.

Epidemics are again a regular part of the news. The genital herpes virus infects half the people in the United States. Chlamydia [a sexually-transmitted disease], virtually unknown until twenty years ago, has become the country's most common infectious disease after the common cold. Germs that used to attack cats, rats, sheep, and monkeys have sickened people from Albuquerque to Moscow. Many forms of cancer are more common, and viruses are implicated in helping to cause several types. Viruses are also suspected of playing roles in chronic fatigue syndrome, Alzheimer's disease, rheumatoid arthritis, systemic lupus, and multiple sclerosis. In recent years, syphilis, tuberculosis, measles, whooping cough, and diphtheria have surfaced not only in poor but in developed nations.

Ignorance a Destructive Luxury

This has all happened with amazing speed—in evolutionary time, during the briefest blink of an eye. The common failure to ask why it has happened reflects a normal tendency toward self-protection. The story of an individual tragedy may grab our attention and threaten our comfort, but we are free to turn our backs when we feel uneasy. News of epidemics and broad biosocial change is different; it brings lingering discomfort. We fear, at the least, an attack of medical student syndrome—the dread, while reading about illness, that one's every inner twitch reflects a malady beyond cure. At the worst, the news makes us imagine cataclysm [disaster], and we want to flee the subject before anxiety or fatalism catches up to us.

Ignorance, however, is a destructive luxury when infections again threaten to take more lives than war and famine. Such a crisis could come during the next fifty years, shaping our lives and our children's. Only by understanding it can we hope to slow and change its course. To reach that understanding requires a fresh look at our relationship with the rest of the living world. . . .

Warnings appeared in the 1950s, when new hemorrhagic fevers broke out in places as far apart as Argentina and India. Hemorrhagic fevers are viral diseases that can cause internal bleeding, shock, and death; the worst are among the deadliest human infections. When the Junin virus first erupted in Argentina, in 1953, it killed up to one-fifth of its victims. In 1955, another fever, only somewhat less lethal, appeared in the Kyasanur Forest region of southwest India. Milder new viral diseases also made debuts, from O'nyong-nyong fever in Uganda, in 1959, to Oropouche in Brazil, in 1961.

These epidemics received little notice in developed nations, but it was different in 1967, when a terrifying new hemorrhagic fever leaped out of Zaire and Sudan. It seized headlines in the West when it struck thirty-one workers in a research laboratory in Marburg, Germany, and killed seven of them. Marburg disease broke out again in Africa in 1976, and its spread remains a threat in the minds of epidemiologists everywhere.

The Apperance of New Diseases

New diseases were also appearing in developed nations. In 1957, a malaria-like infection of cattle called babesiosis turned up in humans in Yugoslavia. It surfaced again in 1969 on Nantucket Island and in the late 1980s in Connecticut; its progress has not ended. In 1968, an unexplained flulike epidemic occurred in Pontiac, Michigan. Almost a decade later it would be recognized as a mild relative of another new illness, Legionnaires' disease.

Far more serious was the growing range and variety of viral encephalitis in the Americas. Many of its victims are children, and those it does not kill may be left blind, deaf, or retarded. Several types of encephalitis are transmitted from birds and wild mammals to people by mosquitoes. In the 1960s, a common new type, LaCrosse encephalitis, was identified, named for the Wisconsin city where the virus was first found. Encephalitis is sporadic, but so dangerous that health agencies monitor it rigorously. Encephalitis viruses and their carriers continue to spread to larger areas, and work and recreation patterns expose more people to the microbes. In 1990, Florida had its worst outbreak in thirty years of one type, St. Louis encephalitis. More than 200 people fell sick there and elsewhere in the United States, and nine died.

When Lassa fever, a horrid new hemorrhagic fever, appeared in Nigeria in 1969, the entire world paid attention. High-speed travel had created a global village for pathogens. Tourists brought the Lassa virus by airplane to Chicago, Toronto, and London, causing scare headlines but only isolated cases. The virus again made news in 1989. A Chicago resident flew to Nigeria for a relative's funeral; he returned and was himself buried two weeks later, killed by the Lassa virus. Like Marburg disease, Lassa fever left health departments around the world watchful and vulnerable.

When Lyme disease, a debilitating tick-borne infection, was identified in 1975, it was not, strictly speaking, new. Scattered cases of a similar ailment had been reported in Europe for many decades, but they remained little more than curiosities. Only in the mid-1970s, in Old Lyme, Connecticut, did the disease become common. Then it increased everywhere. Now it ranges from New England to California, is more frequent in Europe than in North America, and appears on other continents as well. In 1994, it was the most common of all tick-borne and insect-borne diseases in the United States.

Ebola and Swine Flu

When Ebola fever appeared, it made Lyme disease seem trivial. This hemorrhagic fever has death rates of 50 or even 90 percent. After terrifying epidemics in Africa in 1976 and

1979, it seemed to spread no further. Then in 1989 a close relative of Ebola virus turned up in monkeys imported to the United States for medical research. There were no human casualties, but the federal Centers for Disease Control (CDC) issued strict new rules on the importation, quarantine, and handling of primates, which are brought into this country by the tens of thousands each year. So far the African hemorrhagic fevers occur only sporadically outside their native territories, but some may be expanding their ranges. The frightening possibility remains that they could travel and adapt to new hosts in other regions.

In 1976, the first year of Ebola fever, the CDC was worried about a domestic problem as well, a new strain of swine flu virus that might prove to be as lethal as the one that caused the epidemic of 1918. The CDC and drug companies went on an emergency footing to produce a vaccine, and 50 million Americans received shots. The CDC was both relieved and embarrassed when flu remained relatively rare that year, even among those who received no vaccine. However, the shots caused at lease 500 cases of a painful paralytic disorder called Guillain-Barré syndrome. To this day, some people avoid flu shots despite their being at high risk for such flu complications as pneumonia, because of the Guillain-Barré incident.

The swine flu scare gave Americans two warnings. One was that they still had to beware of epidemics with animal reservoirs. The flu virus has many varieties, many reservoirs (such as swine and fowl) that can exchange it, and a spectacular ability to mutate and baffle human immune defenses. The other warning was that medical technologies were creating new ills, some as threatening as chose they were meant to combat.

When a severe respiratory epidemic broke out in Philadelphia in 1976, it was first feared to be swine flu. Many of the victims were American Legionnaires attending a bicentennial-year convention there; hundreds fell ill, and dozens died. Yet no flu virus was found, nor was any other familiar microbe. The mysterious ailment, dubbed Legionnaires' disease, had prominent press coverage for almost six months as researchers sought its cause. They finally found it, a peculiar bacterium that manages to thrive in air conditioners, cooling towers, whirlpool baths, and other pieces hostile to most life forms. Legionellosis still occurs around the world, especially in hospitals and hotels, and recently on a luxury cruise ship. There may be as many as 50,000 cases a year in the United States alone.

The appearance of new infectious diseases was no longer startling in 1980, when toxic shock syndrome (TSS) became epidemic. Hundreds of American women fell gravely ill; some died, and many suffered lasting after-effects. The cause was a toxin produced by a new, probably mutant form of a common bacterium, *Staphylococcus aureus*. TSS was linked to a new type of menstrual tampon, which subsequently was removed from the market, and few cases occurred afterward.

The next decade brought a similar disease, toxic-shock-like syndrome (TSLS). Most people first heard of it in 1990, when it killed Muppeteer Jim Henson. TSLS is extremely virulent and fast-acting; doctors said that starting antibiotic treatment just a few hours earlier might have saved Henson's life. TSLS is caused by type A streptococcus, which usually causes strep throat and scarlet fever. It declined in virulence for almost a century and now has returned in a vicious new form, probably a mutant, in the United States, Europe, and Australia. In 1994, the press made people aware that a fast-acting, supervirulent form of strep A caused "flesh-eating" infections in England and the United States, devouring patients' muscle tissue and killing some of them.

STDs and AIDS

By the 1980s, several new or previously declining types of sexually transmitted diseases (STDs) had become wildfire epidemics. Genital herpes grew from a relatively minor health problem to a national concern. Unlike love, the grim joke says, herpes is forever. This painful, lifelong disease can not only spread to one's sex partners but fatally infect infants as they pass through the birth canal. Herpes increased more than tenfold from the mid-1960s to the mid-1980s; many of its sufferers formed support groups and took oaths of near chastity. They would have been even more frightened had they known that researchers suspected a link between herpes virus and cervical cancer. It turned out that the microbial villain in such cancer is not herpes virus but human papilloma virus (HPV), the cause of genital warts. Like herpes virus, HPV has become rampant. It was only the first of several increasingly wide-spread viruses found to play roles in common types of cancer.

When the AIDS syndrome was identified in 1981, it over-shadowed all other STDs. It is a mass killer without parallel. Only rabies matches its lethal power, but rabies cannot be transmitted from person to person. Even in the best possible scenario—safer sex behavior, effective drugs and vaccines, and constant medical vigilance—AIDS will kill tens of millions of people in the next few decades, leaving entire nations invalids. It is not widely appreciated that viral hepatitis, often transmitted in the same ways as AIDS, sickens and kills even more people around the world each year, and continues to increase at an alarming rate.

As STDs changed and spread, so did more hemorrhagic fevers. A new child killer, dengue shock syndrome, has traveled from Asia to the entire tropical and subtropical world; mosquitoes capable of spreading it have entered the United States. The Seoul hantavirus, which causes Korean hemorrhagic fever, seemed a local problem when it attacked American soldiers in 1950. Then the virus was transported by ship to ports around the world. In 1985, a variety was found in Baltimore harbor rats, and then in Baltimore hospital patients with histories of stroke and kidney disease. Seoul-type viruses are suspected of causing such illnesses everywhere. One of their close cousins, the Four Corners virus that struck in the Southwest in 1993, is also more widespread than was first believed.

The Dance of Survival

Where do these new diseases come from? So far, the only widely publicized answers are those of a few quixotic scientists who point to outer space, and of creationists who blame a vengeful deity. The claims for outer space have a deservedly small following; even some who proffer them do so with tongue in cheek. And many creationists claim just one miracle, the one they believe started the world's clockwork ticking. Some call AIDS a divine chastisement. So far, at least, they have not similarly blamed Lassa fever, Lyme disease, and legionellosis on the sins of Nigerians, suburbanites, and aging veterans.

New diseases do not fall from the sky or leap from some mysterious black box. Parasitism and disease are a natural, in fact necessary, part of life. They are basic to the existence of everything from the earliest, simplest organisms to humans. Diseases, old and new, strike horses, insects, plants, even bacteria. New ones are always coming into existence, most change with time, and some vanish from the earth. A small number of human diseases have always been with us, inherited from our primate ancestors. Chicken pox, for instance, struck the earliest humans, and it remains among us. But most human diseases were once new. They came to us because we changed our environment, our behavior, or both. Sometimes, as is happening now, they came in waves.

Most of these diseases came from other species—smallpox probably from dogs or cattle, hemorrhagic fevers from rodents and monkeys, tuberculosis from cattle and birds, the common cold from horses, AIDS probably from African monkeys. The vehicles by which many reached us were mosquitoes, ticks, and other small creatures that respond quickly to even minimal changes in our shared environment. Some of those changes happened naturally; at least as many we created.

We provide new ecological niches for microbes by tilling fields and domesticating animals, and by bringing into existence gardens and second-growth forests, villages and cities, homes and factories. We give them new homes in discarded truck tires and water tanks, in air conditioners and hospital equipment. We transport them by automobile, ship, and airplane. We alter their opportunities and affect their evolution when we change our abodes, our sex behavior, our diets, our clothing. The faster we change ourselves and our surroundings, the faster new infections reach us. In the past century we have changed the biosphere as much as any glacial surge or meteor impact ever has. So we and microbes are dancing faster than ever in order to survive each other. As we do so, the burdens on our environment and our immune defenses increase.

There is cause for alarm, but not for despair. Our primate ancestors had to cope with new diseases, and so did our Stone Age forebears. So did the first farmers and the first city dwellers. Despite struggles and crises, they were able to survive the challenges. And so, presumably, are we. The human immune system and human imagination are marvels of adaptiveness.

We are in one of those recurring eras of crisis when we accelerate the process of acquiring and adjusting to new pathogens. They, like us, are trying to adapt and survive. Some must be conquered; some require only a wise truce. If we are to adapt and survive, we must start by understanding how we have always coped with new diseases.

Appendix

Excerpts from Original Documents Pertaining to the Black Death

The Appearance and Spread of the Black Death

Document 1: The Black Death Reaches Europe

This is an excerpt from the Historia de Morbo, *by Gabriele de Mussis (died 1356), a lawyer in the Italian city of Piacenza. The work constitutes the most detailed and important primary source for the spread of the Black Death from the Far East to European cities. The author describes the siege of Kaffa (or Caffa), in which the Mongols (Tartars) hurled infected bodies into the Genoese fortress, and local reaction to the arrival of the pestilence in Italy, including parents abandoning children and families torn asunder. Throughout his dramatic narrative, de Mussis heavily emphasizes the notion that the disaster is a divine punishment.*

In 1346, in the countries of the East, countless numbers of Tartars and Saracens [i.e., Muslims] were struck down by a mysterious illness which brought sudden death. Within these countries broad regions, far-spreading provinces, magnificent kingdoms, cities, towns and settlements, ground down by illness and devoured by dreadful death, were soon stripped of their inhabitants. An eastern settlement under the rule of the Tartars called Tana, which lay to the north of Constantinople and was much frequented by Italian merchants, was totally abandoned after an incident there which led to its being besieged and attacked by hordes of Tartars who gathered in a short space of time. The Christian merchants, who had been driven out by force, were so terrified of the power of the Tartars that, to save themselves and their belongings, they fled in an armed ship to Caffa, a settlement in the same part of the world which had been founded long ago by the Genoese.

Oh God! See how the heathen Tartar races, pouring together from all sides, suddenly invested the city of Caffa and besieged the trapped Christians there for almost three years. There, hemmed in by an immense army, they could hardly draw breath, although food could be shipped in, which offered them some hope. But behold, the whole army was affected by a disease which overran the Tartars and killed thousands upon thousands every day. It was as

127

though arrows were raining down from heaven to strike and crush the Tartars' arrogance. All medical advice and attention was useless; the Tartars died as soon as the signs of disease appeared on their bodies: swellings in the armpit or groin caused by coagulating humours, followed by a putrid fever.

The dying Tartars, stunned and stupefied by the immensity of the disaster brought about by the disease, and realising that they had no hope of escape, lost interest in the siege. But they ordered corpses to be placed in catapults and lobbed into the city in the hope that the intolerable stench would kill everyone inside. What seemed like mountains of dead were thrown into the city, and the Christians could not hide or flee or escape from them, although they dumped as many of the bodies as they could in the sea. And soon the rotting corpses tainted the air and poisoned the water supply, and the stench was so overwhelming that hardly one in several thousand was in a position to flee the remains of the Tartar army. Moreover one infected man could carry the poison to others, and infect people and places with the disease by look alone. No one knew, or could discover, a means of defence.

Thus almost everyone who had been in the East, or in the regions to the south and north, fell victim to sudden death after contracting this pestilential disease, as if struck by a lethal arrow which raised a tumour on their bodies. The scale of the mortality and the form which it took persuaded those who lived, weeping and lamenting, through the bitter events of 1346 to 1348—the Chinese, Indians, Persians, Medes, Kurds, Armenians, Cilicians, Georgians, Mesopotamians, Nubians, Ethiopians, Turks, Egyptians, Arabs, Saracens and Greeks (for almost all the East has been affected)—that the last judgement had come.

Now it is time that we passed from east to west, to discuss all the things which we ourselves have seen, or known, or consider likely on the basis of the evidence, and, by so doing, to show forth the terrifying judgements of God. Listen everybody, and it will set tears pouring from your eyes. For the Almighty has said: 'I shall wipe man, whom I created, off the face of the earth. Because he is flesh and blood, let him be turned to dust and ashes. My spirit shall not remain among man.'

—'What are you thinking of, merciful God, thus to destroy your creation and the human race; to order and command its sudden annihilation in this way? What has become of your mercy; the faith of our fathers; the blessed virgin, who holds sinners in her lap; the precious blood of the martyrs; the worthy army of confessors and virgins; the whole host of paradise, who pray ceaselessly for sinners; the most precious death of Christ on the cross and our wonderful redemption? Kind God, I beg that your anger may cease, that you do not destroy sinners in this way, and, because you desire mercy rather than sacrifice, that you turn away all evil from the penitent, and do not allow the just to be condemned with the unjust.'

—'I hear you, sinner, dropping words into my ears. I bid you weep. The time for mercy has passed. I, God, am called to vengeance. It is my pleasure to take revenge on sin and wickedness. I shall give my signs to the dying, let them take steps to provide for the health of their souls.'

As it happened, among those who escaped from Caffa by boat were a few sailors who had been infected with the poisonous disease. Some boats were bound for Genoa, others went to Venice and to other Christian areas. When the sailors reached these places and mixed with the people there, it was as if they had brought evil spirits with them: every city, every settlement, every place was poisoned by the contagious pestilence, and their inhabitants, both men and women, died suddenly. And when one person had contracted the illness, he poisoned his whole family even as he fell and died, so that those preparing to bury his body were seized by death in the same way. Thus death entered through the windows, and as cities and towns were depopulated their inhabitants mourned their dead neighbours.

—Speak, Genoa, of what you have done. Describe, Sicily and Isole Pelagie, the judgements of God. Recount, Venice, Tuscany and the whole of Italy, what you have done.

—We Genoese and Venetians bear the responsibility for revealing the judgements of God. Alas, once our ships had brought us to port we went to our homes. And because we had been delayed by tragic events, and because among us there were scarcely ten survivors from a thousand sailors, relations, kinsmen and neighbours flocked to us from all sides. But, to our anguish, we were carrying the darts of death. While they hugged and kissed us we were spreading poison from our lips even as we spoke.

When they returned to their own folk, these people speedily poisoned the whole family, and within three days the afflicted family would succumb to the dart of death. Mass funerals had to be held and there was not enough room to bury the growing numbers of dead. Priests and doctors, upon whom most of the care of the sick devolved, had their hands full in visiting the sick and, alas, by the time they left they too had been infected and followed the dead immediately to the grave. Oh fathers! Oh mothers! Oh children and wives! For a long time prosperity preserved you from harm, but one grave now covers you and the unfortunate alike. You who enjoyed the world and upon whom pleasure and prosperity smiled, who mingled joys with follies, the same tomb receives you and you are handed over as food for worms. Oh hard death, impious death, bitter death, cruel death, who divides parents, divorces spouses, parts children, separates brothers and sisters. We bewail our wretched plight. The past has devoured us, the present is gnawing our entrails, the future threatens yet greater dangers. What we laboured to amass with feverish activity, we have lost in one hour.

Where are the fine clothes of gilded youth? Where is nobility and the courage of fighters, where the mature wisdom of elders and the regal throng of great ladies, where the piles of treasure and precious stones? Alas! All have been destroyed; thrust aside by death. To whom shall we turn, who can help us? To flee is impossible, to hide futile. Cities, fortresses, fields, woods, highways and rivers are ringed by thieves—which is to say by evil spirits, the executioners of the supreme Judge, preparing endless punishments for us all.

We can unfold a terrifying event which happened when an army was camped near Genoa. Four of the soldiers left the force in search of plunder and made their way to Rivarolo on the coast, where the disease had killed all the inhabitants. Finding the houses shut up, and no one about, they broke into one of the houses and stole a fleece which they found on a bed. They then rejoined the army and on the following night the four of them bedded down under the fleece. When morning comes it finds them dead. As a result everyone panicked, and thereafter nobody would use the goods and clothes of the dead, or even handle them, but rejected them outright.

Scarcely one in seven of the Genoese survived. In Venice, where an inquiry was held into the mortality, it was found that more than 70% of the people had died, and that within a short period 20 out of 24 excellent physicians had died. The rest of Italy, Sicily and Apulia and the neighbouring regions maintain that they have been virtually emptied of inhabitants. The people of Florence, Pisa and Lucca, finding themselves bereft of their fellow residents, emphasise their losses. The Roman Curia at Avignon, the provinces on both sides of the Rhône, Spain, France, and the Empire cry up their griefs and disasters—all of which makes it extraordinarily difficult for me to give an accurate picture.

By contrast, what befell the Saracens can be established from trustworthy accounts. In the city of Babylon alone (the heart of the Sultan's power), 480,000 of his subjects are said to have been carried off by disease in less than three months in 1348—and this is known from the Sultan's register which records the names of the dead, because he receives a gold bezant for each person buried. I am silent about Damascus and his other cities, where the number of dead was infinite. In the other countries of the East, which are so vast that it takes three years to ride across them and which have a population of 10,000 for every one inhabitant of the west, it is credibly reported that countless people have died.

Everyone has a responsibility to keep some record of the disease and the deaths, and because I am myself from Piacenza I have been urged to write more about what happened there in 1348. Some Genoese, whom the disease had forced to flee, crossed the Alps in search of a safe place to live and so came to Lombardy. Some had merchandise with them and sold it while they were staying in Bobbio, whereupon the purchaser, their host, and his whole household, together with several neighbours, were infected and died suddenly of the disease. One man there, wanting to make his will, died along with the notary, the priest who heard his confession, and the people summoned to witness the will, and they were all buried together on the following day. The scale of the disaster was such that virtually all the inhabitants were subsequently struck down by sudden death and only a tiny handful remained alive.

Another of the Genoese, who was already suffering from the illness, managed to reach Piacenza. Finding himself unwell, he sought out his close friend Fulco della Croce, who gave him shelter. He immediately took to his bed and died, and then straightaway Fulco, with his whole household and many of the neighbours, died too. And that, briefly, is how this disease (spreading rapidly throughout the world) arrived in Piacenza. I don't know where to begin. Cries and laments arise on all sides. Day after day one sees the Cross and the Host being carried about the city, and countless dead being buried. The ensuing mortality was so great that people could scarcely snatch breath. The living made preparations for their burial, and because there was not enough room for individual graves, pits had to be dug in colonnades and piazzas, where nobody had ever been buried before. It often happened that man and wife, father and son, mother and daughter, and soon the whole household and many neighbours, were buried together in one place. The same thing happened in Castell' Arquato and

Viguzzolo and in the other towns, villages, cities and settlements, and last of all in the Val Tidone, where they had hitherto escaped the plague.

Very many people died. One Oberto de Sasso, who had come from the infected neighbourhood around the church of the Franciscans, wished to make his will and accordingly summoned a notary and his neighbours as witnesses, all of whom, more than sixty of them, died soon after. At this time the Dominican friar Syfredo de Bardis, a man of prudence and great learning who had visited the Holy Sepulchre, also died, along with 23 brothers of the same house. There also died within a short time the Franciscan friar Bertolino Coxadocha of Piacenza, renowned for his learning and many virtues, along with 24 brothers of the same house, nine of them on one day; seven of the Augustinians; the Carmelite friar Francesco Todischi with six of his brethren; four of the order of Mary; more than sixty prelates and parish priests from the city and district of Piacenza; many nobles; countless young people; numberless women, particularly those who were pregnant. It is too distressing to recite any more, or to lay bare the wounds inflicted by so great a disaster.

Let all creation tremble with fear before the judgement of God. Let human frailty submit to its creator. May a greater grief be kindled in all hearts, and tears well up in all eyes as future ages hear what happened in this disaster. When one person lay sick in a house no one would come near. Even dear friends would hide themselves away, weeping. The physician would not visit. The priest, panic-stricken, administered the sacraments with fear and trembling.

Listen to the tearful voices of the sick: 'Have pity, have pity, my friends. At least say something, now that the hand of God has touched me.'

'Oh father, why have you abandoned me? Do you forget that I am your child?'

'Mother, where have you gone? Why are you now so cruel to me when only yesterday you were so kind? You fed me at your breast and carried me within your womb for nine months.'

'My children, whom I brought up with toil and sweat, why have you run away?'

Man and wife reached out to each other, 'Alas, once we slept happily together but now are separated and wretched.'

And when the sick were in the throes of death, they still called out piteously to their family and neighbours, 'Come here. I'm thirsty, bring me a drink of water. I'm still alive. Don't be frightened. Perhaps I won't die. Please hold me tight, hug my wasted body. You ought to be holding me in your arms.'

At this, as everyone else kept their distance, somebody might take pity and leave a candle burning by the bed head as he fled. And when the victim had breathed his last, it was often the mother who shrouded her son and placed him in the coffin, or the husband who did the same for his wife, for everybody else refused to touch the dead body. No prayer, trumpet or bell summoned friends and neighbours to the funeral, nor was mass performed. Degraded and poverty-striken wretches were paid to carry the great and noble to burial, for the social equals of the dead person dared not attend the funeral for fear of being struck down themselves. Men were borne to burial by day and night, since needs must, and with only a short service. In many cases the houses of the dead had to be shut up, for no one dared enter them or touch the belongings of the dead. No one knew what to do. Everyone, one by one, fell in turn to death's dart.

What a tragic and wretched sight! Who would not shed sympathetic tears? Who would not be shaken by the disastrous plague and the terrors of death? But our hearts have grown hard now that we have no future to look forward to. Alas. Our inheritance has been diverted to strangers, our homes to outsiders. It is only the survivors who can enjoy the relief of tears.

I am overwhelmed, I can't go on. Everywhere one turns there is death and bitterness to be described. The hand of the Almighty strikes repeatedly, to greater and greater effect. The terrible judgement gains in power as time goes by.

—What shall we do? Kind Jesus, receive the souls of the dead, avert your gaze from our sins and blot out all our iniquities.

From *The Black Death*, by Rosemary Horrox (Manchester, UK: Manchester University Press, 1994). Reprinted by permission of the publisher.

Document 2: The Epidemic Strikes Florence

The great fourteenth-century Italian writer Giovanni Boccaccio left behind a long, detailed, and graphic depiction of the onset of the Black Death in Florence, Italy, in the introduction to his famous collection of tales, The Decameron. *About half of that introduction is reproduced below. Boccaccio begins with a disclaimer, apologizing to his readers for opening his book with a description of the dreadful plague, but insisting that it is necessary to understanding the rest of his tales. He then describes the symptoms of the disease and conjectures (incorrectly) that it spreads di-*

rectly from person to person. He also tells how people reacted to the disaster (locking themselves in their houses, fleeing, and so on) and, like de Mussis, relates how relatives and friends abandoned one another.

Whenever, most gracious ladies, I consider how compassionate you are by nature, I realize that in your judgment the present work will seem to have had a serious and painful beginning, for it recalls in its opening the unhappy memory of the deadly plague just passed, dreadful and pitiful to all those who saw or heard about it. But I do not wish to frighten you away from reading any further, by giving you the impression that all you are going to do is spend your time sighing and weeping while you read. This horrible beginning will be like the ascent of a steep and rough mountainside, beyond which there lies a most beautiful and delightful plain, and the degree of pleasure derived by the climbers will be in proportion to the difficulty of the climb and the descent. And just as pain is the extreme limit of pleasure, so, then, misery ends with unanticipated happiness. This brief pain (I say brief since it contains few words) will be quickly followed by the sweetness and the delight which I promised you before, and which, had I not promised, might not be expected from such a beginning. To tell the truth, if I could have conveniently led you by any other way than this, which I know is a bitter one, I would have gladly done so; but since it is otherwise impossible to demonstrate how the stories you are about to read came to be told, I am obliged, as it were, by necessity to write about it this way.

Let me say, then, that thirteen hundred and forty-eight years had already passed after the fruitful Incarnation of the Son of God when into the distinguished city of Florence, more noble than any other Italian city, there came a deadly pestilence. Either because of the influence of heavenly bodies or because of God's just wrath as a punishment to mortals for our wicked deeds, the pestilence, originating some years earlier in the East, killed an infinite number of people as it spread relentlessly from one place to another until finally it had stretched its miserable length all over the West. And against this pestilence no human wisdom or foresight was of any avail; quantities of filth were removed from the city by officials charged with the task; the entry of any sick person into the city was prohibited; and many directives were issued concerning the maintenance of good health. Nor were the humble supplications rendered not once but many times by the pious to God, through public processions or by other means, in any way efficacious; for almost at the beginning of springtime of the year in question the plague began to show its sorrowful effects in an extraordinary manner. It did not assume the form it had in the East, where bleeding from the nose was a manifest sign of inevitable death, but rather it showed its first signs in men and women alike by means of swellings either in the groin or under the armpits, some of which grew to the size of an ordinary apple and others to the size of an egg (more or less), and the people called them *gavoccioli* [buboes]. And from the two parts of the body already mentioned, in very little time, the said deadly *gavoccioli* began to spread indiscriminately over every part of the body; then, after this, the symptoms of the illness changed to black or livid spots appearing on the arms and thighs, and on every part of the body—sometimes there were large ones and other times a number of little ones scattered all around. And just as the *gavoccioli* were originally, and still are, a very definite indication of impending death, in like manner these spots came to mean the same thing for whoever contracted them. Neither a doctor's advice nor the strength of medicine could do anything to cure this illness; on the contrary, either the nature of the illness was such that it afforded no cure, or else the doctors were so ignorant that they did not recognize its cause and, as a result, could not prescribe the proper remedy (in fact, the number of doctors, other than the well-trained, was increased by a large number of men and women who had never had any medical training); at any rate, few of the sick were ever cured, and almost all died after the third day of the appearance of the previously described symptoms (some sooner, others later), and most of them died without fever or any other side effects.

This pestilence was so powerful that it was transmitted to the healthy by contact with the sick, the way a fire close to dry or oily things will set them aflame. And the evil of the plague went even further: not only did talking to or being around the sick bring infection and a common death, but also touching the clothes of the sick or anything touched or used by them seemed to communicate this very disease to the person involved. What I am about to say is incredible to hear, and if I and others had not witnessed it with our own eyes, I should not dare believe it (let alone write about it), no matter how trustworthy a person I might have heard it from. Let me say, then, that the plague described here was of such virulence in spreading from one person to another that not only did it pass from one man to the next, but, what's more, it was often transmitted from the garments of a sick or dead man to animals that not only became contaminated by the disease but also died within a brief period of time. My own eyes, as I said earlier, were witness to such a thing one day: when the rags of a poor man who died of this disease were thrown into the public street, two pigs came upon them, and, as they are wont to do, first with their snouts and then with their teeth they took the rags and shook them around; and within a short time, after a number of convulsions, both pigs fell dead upon the ill-fated rags, as if they had been poisoned. From these and many similar or worse occurrences there came about such fear and such fantastic notions among those who remained alive that almost all of them took a very cruel attitude in the matter; that is, they completely avoided the sick and their possessions, and in so doing, each one believed that he was protecting his own good health.

There were some people who thought that living moderately and avoiding any excess might help a great deal in resisting this disease, and so they gathered in small groups and lived entirely apart from everyone else. They shut themselves up in those houses where there were no sick people and where one could live well by eating the most delicate of foods and drinking the finest of wines (doing so always in moderation), allowing no one to speak about or listen to anything said about the sick and the dead outside; these people lived, entertaining themselves with music and other pleasures that they could arrange. Others thought the opposite: they believed that drinking excessively, enjoying life, going about singing and celebrating, satisfying in every way the appetites as best one could, laughing, and making light of everything that happened was the best medicine for such a disease; so they practiced to the fullest what they believed by going from one tavern to another all day and night, drinking to excess; and they would often make merry in private homes, doing everything that pleased or amused them the most. This they were able to do easily, for everyone felt he was doomed to die and, as a result, abandoned his property, so that most of the houses had become common property, and any stranger who came upon them used them as if he were their rightful owner. In addition to this bestial behavior, they always managed to avoid the sick as best they could. And in this great affliction and misery of our city the revered authority of the laws, both divine and human, had fallen and almost completely disappeared, for, like other men, the ministers and executors of the laws were either dead or sick or so short of help that it was impossible for them to fulfill their duties; as a result, everybody was free to do as he pleased.

Many others adopted a middle course between the two attitudes just described: neither did they restrict their food or drink so much as the first group nor did they fall into such dissoluteness and drunkenness as the second; rather, they satisfied their appetites to a moderate degree. They did not shut themselves up, but went around carrying in their hands flowers, or sweet-smelling herbs, or various kinds of spices; and they would often put these things to their noses, believing that such smells were a wonderful means of purifying the brain, for all the air seemed infected with the stench of dead bodies, sickness, and medicines.

Others were of a crueler opinion (though it was, perhaps, a safer one): they maintained that there was no better medicine against the plague than to flee from it; convinced of this reasoning and caring only about themselves, men and women in great numbers abandoned their city, their houses, their farms, their relatives, and their possessions and sought other places, going at least as far away as the Florentine countryside—as if the wrath of God could not pursue them with this pestilence wherever they went but would only strike those it found within the walls of the city! Or perhaps they thought that Florence's last hour had come and that no one in the city would remain alive.

And not all those who adopted these diverse opinions died, nor did they all escape with their lives; on the contrary, many of those who thought this way were falling sick everywhere, and since they had given, when they were healthy, the bad example of avoiding the sick, they in turn were abandoned and left to languish away without any care. The fact was that one citizen avoided another, that almost no one cared for his neighbor, and that relatives rarely or hardly ever visited each other—they stayed far apart. This disaster had struck such fear into the hearts of men and women that brother abandoned brother, uncle abandoned nephew, sister left brother, and very often wife abandoned husband, and—even worse, almost unbelievable—fathers and mothers neglected to tend and care for their children as if they were not their own.

Thus, for the countless multitude of men and women who fell sick, there remained no support except the charity of their friends (and these were few) or the greed of servants, who worked for inflated salaries without regard to the service they performed and who, in spite of this, were few and far between; and those few were men or women of little wit (most of them not trained for such service) who did little else but hand different things to the sick when requested to do so or watch over them while they died, and in this service, they very often lost their own lives and their profits. And since the sick were abandoned by their neighbors, their parents, and their friends and there was a scarcity of servants, a practice that was previously almost unheard of spread through the city: when a woman fell sick, no matter how attractive or beautiful or noble she might be, she did not mind having a manservant (whoever he might be, no matter how young or old he was), and she had no shame whatsoever in revealing any part of her body to him—the way she would have done to a woman—when necessity of her sickness required her to do so. This practice was, perhaps, in the days that followed the pestilence, the cause of looser morals in the women who survived the plague. And so, many people died who, by chance, might have survived if they had been attended to. Between the lack of competent attendants that the sick were unable to obtain and the violence of the pestilence itself, so many, many people died in the city both day and night that it was incredible just to hear this described, not to mention seeing it! Therefore, out of sheer necessity, there arose among those who remained alive customs which were contrary to the established practices of the time.

It was the custom, as it is again today, for the women relatives and neighbors to gather together in the house of a dead person and there to mourn with the women who had been dearest to him; on the other hand, in front of the deceased's home, his male relatives would gather together with his male neighbors and other citizens, and the clergy also came, many of them or sometimes just a few, depending upon the social class of the dead man. Then, upon the shoulders of his equals, he was carried to the church chosen by him before death with the funeral pomp of candles and chants. With the fury of the pestilence increasing, this custom, for the most part, died out and other practices took its place. And so not only did people die without having a number of women around them, but there were many who passed away without having even a single witness present, and very few were granted the piteous laments and bitter tears of their relatives; on the contrary, most relatives were somewhere else, laughing, joking, and amusing themselves; even the women learned this practice too well, having put aside, for the most part, their womanly compassion for their own safety. Very few were the dead whose bodies were accompanied to the church by more than ten or twelve of their neighbors, and these dead bodies were not even carried on the shoulders of honored and reputable citizens but rather by gravediggers from the lower classes that were called *becchini*. Working for pay, they would pick up the bier and hurry it off, not to the church the dead man had chosen before his death but, in most cases, to the church closest by, accompanied by four or six churchmen with just a few candles, and often none at all. With the help of these *becchini*, the churchmen would place the body as fast as they could in whatever unoccupied grave they could find without going to the trouble of saying long or solemn burial services.

The plight of the lower class and, perhaps, a large part of the middle class was even more pathetic: most of them stayed in their homes or neighborhoods either because of their poverty or because of their hopes for remaining safe, and every day they fell sick by the thousands; and not having servants or attendants of any kind, they almost always died. Many ended their lives in the public streets, during the day or at night, while many others who died in their homes were discovered dead by their neighbors only by the smell of their decomposing bodies. The city was full of corpses. The dead were usually given the same treatment by their neighbors, who were moved more by the fear that the decomposing corpses would contaminate them than by any charity they might have felt toward the deceased: either by themselves or with the assistance of porters (when they were available), they would drag the corpse out of the home and place it in front of the doorstep, where, usually in the morning, quantities of dead bodies could be seen by any passerby; then they were laid out on biers, or for lack of biers, on a plank. Nor did a bier carry only one corpse; sometimes it was used for two or three at a time. More than once, a single bier would serve for a wife and husband, two or three brothers, a father or son, or other relatives, all at the same time. And very often it happened that two priests, each with a cross, would be on their way to bury someone, when porters carrying three or four biers would just follow along behind them; and whereas these priests thought they had just one dead man to bury, they had, in fact, six or eight and sometimes more. Moreover, the dead were honored with no tears or candles or funeral mourners; in fact, things had reached such a point that the people who died were cared for as we care for goats today. Thus it became quite obvious that the very thing which in normal times wise men had not been able to resign themselves to, even though then it struck seldom and less harshly, became as a result of this colossal misfortune a matter of indifference to even the most simpleminded people.

So many corpses would arrive in front of a church every day and at every hour that the amount of holy ground for burials was certainly insufficient for the ancient custom of giving each body its individual place; when all the graves were full, huge trenches were dug in all of the cemeteries of the churches and into them the new arrivals were dumped by the hundreds; and they were packed in there with dirt, one on top of another, like a ship's cargo, until the trench was filled.

But instead of going over every detail of the past miseries which befell our city, let me say that the hostile winds blowing there did not, however, spare the surrounding countryside any evil; there, not to speak of the towns which, on a smaller scale, were like the city, in the scattered villages and in the fields the poor, miserable peasants and their families, without any medical assistance or aid of servants, died on the roads and in their fields and in their homes, as many by day as by night, and they died not like men but more like animals. Because of this they, like the city dwellers, became careless in their ways and did not look after their possessions or their businesses; furthermore, when they saw that death was upon them, completely neglecting the future fruits of their past labors, their livestock, their property, they did their best to consume what they already had at hand. So it came about that oxen, donkeys, sheep, pigs, chickens, and even dogs, man's most faithful companion, were driven from their homes into the fields, where the wheat was left not only unharvested but also unreaped, and they were allowed to roam where they wished; and many of these animals, almost as if they were rational beings, returned at night to their homes without any guidance from a shepherd, full after a good day's meal. . . .

Oh, how many great palaces, beautiful homes, and noble dwellings, once filled with families, gentlemen, and ladies, were now emptied, down to the last servant! How many notable families, vast domains, and famous fortunes remained without legitimate heir! How many valiant men, beautiful women, and charming young boys, who might have been pronounced very healthy by Galen, Hippocrates, and Aesculapius (not to mention lesser physicians), ate breakfast in the morning with their relatives, companions, and friends and then in the evening dined with their ancestors in the other world!

Giovanni Boccaccio, *The Decameron*, trans. Mark Musa and Peter Bondanella. New York: W.W. Norton, 1982, pp. 5–12.

Document 3: The Plague in Siena

Like Florence, Venice, and other populous northern Italian cities, Siena suffered greatly under the Black Death's onslaught. This excerpt from the chronicle of the contemporary Sienese notable Agnolo de Tura del Grasso, nicknamed "the Fat," is important for its attention to specific mortality figures, rather than generalities, such as "many" or "over half the population" died. Scholars believe that del Grasso consulted government archives and other public records, suggesting that his figures may be reasonably accurate.

The mortality began in Siena in May [1348]. It was a cruel and horrible thing; and I do not know where to begin to tell of the cruelty and the pitiless ways. It seemed to almost everyone that one became stupified by seeing the pain. And it is impossible for the human tongue to recount the awful thing. Indeed one who did not see such horribleness can be called blessed. And the victims died almost immediately. They would swell beneath their armpits and in their groins, and fall over dead while talking. Father abandoned child, wife husband, one brother another; for this illness seemed to strike through the breath and sight. And so they died. And none could be found to bury the dead for money or friendship. Members of a household brought their dead to a ditch as best they could, without priest, without divine offices. Nor did the death bell sound. And in many places in Siena great pits were dug and piled deep with the multitude of dead. And they died by the hundreds both day and night, and all were thrown in those ditches and covered over with earth. And as soon as those ditches were filled more were dug.

And I, Agnolo di Tura, called the Fat, buried my five children with my own hands. And there were also those who were so sparsely covered with earth that the dogs dragged them forth and devoured many bodies throughout the city. There was no one who wept for any death, for all awaited death. And so many died that all believed that it was the end of the world. And no medicine or any other defense availed. And the lords selected three citizens who received a thousand gold florins from the commune of Siena that they were to spend on the poor sick and to bury the poor dead. And it was all so horrible that I, the writer, cannot think of it and so will not continue. This situation continued until September, and it would take too long to write of it. And it is found that at this time there died in Siena 36,000 persons twenty years of age or less, and the aged and other people [died], to a total of 52,000 in all in Siena. And in the suburbs of Siena 28,000 persons died; so that in all it is found that in the city and suburbs of Siena 80,000 persons died. Thus at this time Siena and its suburbs had more than 30,000 men, and there remained in Siena [alone] less than 10,000 men. And those that survived were like persons distraught and almost without feeling. And many walls and other things were abandoned, and all the mines of silver and gold and copper that existed in Sienese territory were abandoned as is seen; for in the countryside (contado) many more people died, many lands and villages were abandoned, and no one remained there. I will not write of the cruelty that there was in the countryside, of the wolves and wild beasts that ate the poorly buried corpses, and of other cruelties that would be too painful to those who read of them. . . .

The city of Siena seemed almost uninhabited for almost no one was found in the city. And then, when the pestilence abated, all who survived gave themselves over to pleasures: monks, priests, nuns, and lay men and women all enjoyed themselves, and none worried about spending and gambling. And everyone thought himself rich because he had escaped and regained the world, and no one knew how to allow himself to do nothing. . . .

At this time in Siena the great and noble project of enlarging the cathedral of Siena that had been begun a few years earlier was abandoned. . . .

After the pestilence the Sienese appointed two judges and three non-Sienese notaries whose task it was to handle the wills that had been made at that time. And so they searched them out and found them. . . .

1349. After the great pestilence of the past year each person lived according to his own caprice, and everyone tended to seek pleasure in eating and drinking, hunting, catching birds, and gaming. And all money had fallen into the hands of *nouveaux riches* ["newly rich," usually those who had profited by confiscating the land abandoned by plague victims].

Quoted in William M. Bowsky, *The Black Death: A Turning Point in History?* New York: Holt, Rhinehart and Winston, 1971, pp. 13–14.

Document 4: Padua Devastated

Padua, in northeastern Italy, and its immediate environs sustained losses of about a third of the population during the great epidemic, according to this excerpt from an old Italian chronicle of the region. This is in keeping with modern estimates of the death toll in most European regions. Significantly, the chronicle mentions the imposition of travel bans to other cities, an early, though fruitless, attempt by local government to fight the pestilence, and also the fact that large numbers of doctors were stricken and died along with patients.

Almighty God, who does not desire the death of a sinner, but that he may be converted and live, first threatens and secondly strikes to reform the human race, not to destroy it. Wishing to assail the human race with enormous and unprecedented blows, his terrifying judgement began firstly in the furthest part of the world, in the countries of the East. After he had struck at the Tartars, Turks and all the other unbelievers, there was on 25 January 1348, at the 23rd hour, a great earthquake to terrify the Christians, which lasted for half an hour. After which the unprecedented plague crossed the sea and so came to the Veneto, Lombardy, the March, Tuscany, Germany, France and spread through virtually the whole world. It was carried by some infected people who had travelled from the East and who, by sight alone, or by touch, or by breathing on them, killed everyone. The infection was incurable; it could not be avoided. The wife fled the embrace of a dear husband, the father that of a son, and the brother that of a brother. Even the houses or clothes of the victims could kill. Those burying, carrying, seeing or touching the infected often died suddenly themselves. Just as one infected sheep infects the whole flock, so one death within a household was always followed by the death of all the rest, right down to the dogs. The bodies even of noblemen lay unburied. Many, at a price, were buried by poor wretches, without priests or candles. Indeed in Venice, where 100,000 died, boats were hired at great expense to carry bodies to the islands and the city was virtually deserted.

A single stranger carried the infection to Padua, to such effect that perhaps a third of the people died within the region as a whole. In the hope of avoiding such a plague, cities banned the entry of all outsiders, with the result that merchants were unable to travel from city to city. Cities and settlements were left desolate by this calamity. No voices could be heard, except in mourning and lamentation. The voice of the bride and groom ceased, and so did music, the songs of young people and all rejoicing. The plagues in the days of Pharoah, David, Ezechiel and Pope Gregory now seemed nothing by comparison, for this plague encircled the whole globe. In the days of Noah God did not destroy all living souls and it was possible for the human race to recover.

As described above, some were infected very badly by this plague and died suddenly from blood poisoning, others from a malignant tumour, or from worms. A certain sign of death, found on almost everyone, were incurable tumours near the genitals, or under the armpits, or in some other part of the body, accompanied by deadly fevers. People with these died on the first or second day; after the third day, although rarely, there was some hope of recovery. Some people fell asleep and never woke up, but passed away. Doctors frankly confessed that they had no cure for the plague, and the most accomplished of them died of it. During the plague Guerra Sambonifacio, *podestà* of Siena, died with virtually all his household. There was also terrible mortality at Florence, Pisa and throughout the whole of Tuscany. The plague generally lasted for six months after its outbreak in each area. The noble man Andrea Morosini, *podestà* of Padua, died in July in his third term of office. His son was put in office, but died immediately. Note, however, that amazingly during this plague no king, prince, or ruler of a city died.

From *The Black Death*, by Rosemary Horrox (Manchester, UK: Manchester University Press, 1994). Reprinted by permission of the publisher.

Document 5: The Black Death Spreads to England

In this contemporary description of the Black Death, fourteenth-century English chronicler Henry Knighton suggests that the contagion first entered England at Southampton. This differs from other early English accounts, which name Bristol, Melcombe, and other towns as the first to feel the plague's wrath. Like other accounts, however, Knighton associates earthquakes with the epidemic. He also mentions large numbers of sheep dying from disease, which is inconsistent with bubonic plague and has been cited as evidence that the Black Death may have been one or more other diseases. Knighton's narrative is also valuable for recording the economic impact of the disaster, including sharp rises in labor costs.

In this year [1348] and in the following one there was a general mortality of men throughout the whole world. It first began in India, then in Tharsis [Taurus?], then it came to the Saracens [i.e., Muslims], and finally to the Christians and Jews, so that in the space of one year, from Easter to Easter, as the rumour spread in the Roman curia, there had died, as if by sudden death, in those remote regions eight thousand legions, besides the Christians. The king of Tharsis, seeing such a sudden and unheard-of slaughter of his people, began a journey to Avignon with a great multitude of his nobles, to propose to the pope that he would become a Christian and be baptized by him, thinking that he might thus mitigate the vengeance of God upon his people because of their wicked unbelief. Then, when he had journeyed for twenty days, he heard that the pestilence had struck among the Christians, just as among other peoples. So, turning in his tracks, he travelled no farther but hastened to return home. The Christians, pursuing these people from behind, slew about seven thousand of them.

There died in Avignon in one day one thousand three hundred and twelve persons, according to a count made for the pope, and, another day, four hundred persons and more. Three hundred and fifty-eight of the Friars Preachers in the region of Provence died during Lent. At Montpellier, there remained out of a hundred and forty friars only seven. There were left at Magdalena only seven friars out of a hundred and sixty, and yet enough. At Marseilles, of a hundred and fifty Friars Minor, there remained only one who could tell the others, that was well, indeed. Of the Carmelites, more than a hundred and sixty-six had died at Avignon before the citizens found out what had happened. For they believed that one had killed another. There was not one of the English Hermits left in Avignon. . . .

At this same time the pestilence became prevalent in England, beginning in the autumn in certain places. It spread throughout the land, ending in the same season of the following year. At the same time many cities in Corinth and Achaia were overturned, and the earth swallowed them. Castles and fortresses were broken, laid low, and swallowed up. Mountains in Cyprus were levelled into one, so that the flow of the rivers was impeded, and many cities were submerged and villages destroyed. Similarly, when a certain friar was preaching at Naples, the whole city was destroyed by an earthquake. Suddenly, the earth was opened up, as if a stone had been thrown into water, and everyone died along with the preaching friar, except for one friar who, fleeing, escaped into a garden outside the city. All of these things were done by an earthquake. . . .

Then that most grievous pestilence penetrated the coastal regions [of England] by way of Southampton, and came to Bristol, and people died as if the whole strength of the city were seized by sudden dentin. For there were few who lay in their beds more than three days or two and a half days; then that savage death snatched them about the second day. In Leicester, in the little parish of St. Leonard, more than three hundred and eighty died; in the parish of the Holy Cross, more than four hundred, and in the parish of St. Margaret in Leicester, more than seven hundred. And so in each parish, they died in great numbers. Then the bishop of Lincoln sent through the whole diocese, and gave the general power to each and every priest, both regular and secular, to hear confessions and to absolve, by the full and entire power of the bishop, except only in the case of debt. And they might absolve in that case if satisfaction could be made by the person while he lived, or from his property after his death. Likewise, the pope granted full remission of all sins, to be absolved completely, to anyone who was in danger of death, and he granted this power to last until the following Easter. And everyone was allowed to choose his confessor as he pleased.

During this same year, there was a great mortality of sheep everywhere in the kingdom; in one place and in one pasture, more than five thousand sheep died and became so putrefied that neither beast nor bird wanted to touch them. And the price of everything was cheap, because of the fear of death; there were very few who took any care for their wealth, or for anything else. For a man could buy a horse for half a mark, which before was worth forty shillings, a large fat ox for four shillings, a cow for twelve pence, a heifer for sixpence, a large fat sheep for four pence, a sheep for threepence, a lamb for two pence, a fat pig for five pence, a stone of wool for nine pence. And the sheep and cattle wandered about through the fields and among the crops, and there was no one to go after them or to collect them. They perished in countless numbers everywhere, in secluded ditches and hedges, for lack of watching, since there was such a lack of serfs and servants, that no one knew what he should do. For there is no memory of a mortality so severe and so savage from the time of Vortigern, king of the Britons, in whose time, as Bede [an early medieval chronicler] says, the living did not suffice to bury the dead. In the following autumn, one could not hire a reaper at a lower wage than eight pence with food, or a mower at less than twelve pence with food. Because of this, much grain rotted in the fields for lack of harvesting, but in the year of the plague, as was said above, among other things there was so great an abundance of all kinds of grain that no one seemed to have concerned himself about it.

The Scots, hearing of the cruel pestilence in England, suspected that this had come upon the English by the avenging hand of God, and when they wished to swear an oath, they swore this one, as the vulgar rumour reached the ears of the English, "be the foul deth of Engelond." And so the Scots, believing that the horrible vengeance of God had fallen on the English, came together in the forest of Selkirk to plan an invasion of the whole kingdom of England. But savage mortality supervened, and the sudden and frightful cruelty of death struck the Scots. In a short time, about five thousand died; the rest, indeed, both sick and well, prepared to return home, but the English, pursuing them, caught up with them, and slew a great many of them.

Master Thomas Bradwardine was consecrated archbishop of Canterbury by the pope, and when he returned to England, came to London. In less than two days he was dead. He was famous above all other clerks in Christendom, in theology especially, but also in other liberal studies. At this same time there was so great a lack of priests everywhere that many widowed churches had no divine services, no masses, matins, vespers, sacraments, and sacramentals. One could hardly hire a chaplain to minister to any church for less than ten pounds or ten marks, and whereas, before the pestilence, when there were plenty of priests, one could hire a chaplain for five or four marks or for two marks, with board, there was scarcely anyone at this time who wanted to accept a position for twenty pounds or twenty marks. But within a short time a very great multitude whose wives had died of the plague rushed into holy orders. Of these many were illiterate and, it seemed, simply laymen who knew nothing except how to read to some extent. The hides of cattle went up from a low price to twelve pence, and for shoes the price went to ten, twelve, fourteen pence; for a pair of leggings, to three and four shillings.

Meanwhile, the king ordered chat in every county of the kingdom, reapers and other labourers should not receive more than they were accustomed to receive, under the penalty provided in the statute, and he renewed the statute from this time. The labourers, however, were so arrogant and hostile that they did not heed the king's command, but if anyone wished to hire them, he had to pay them what they wanted, and either lose his fruits and crops or satisfy the arrogant and greedy desire of the labourers as they wished. When it was made known to the king that they had not obeyed his mandate, and had paid higher wages to the labourers, he imposed heavy fines on the abbots, the priors, the great lords and the lesser ones, and on others both greater and lesser in the kingdom. From certain ones he took a hundred shillings, from some, forty shillings, from others, twenty shillings, and from each according to what he could pay. And he took from each ploughland in the whole kingdom twenty shillings, and not one-fifteenth less than this. Then the king had many labourers arrested, and put them in prison. Many such hid themselves and ran away to the forests and woods for a while, and those who were captured were heavily fined. And the greater number swore that they would not take daily wages above those set by ancient custom, and so they were freed from prison. It was done in like manner concerning other artisans in towns and villages. . . .

After the aforesaid pestilence, many buildings, both large and small, in all cities, towns, and villages had collapsed, and had completely fallen to the ground in the absence of inhabitants. Likewise, many small villages and hamlets were completely deserted; there was not one house left in them, but all those who had lived in them were dead. It is likely that many such hamlets will never again be inhabited. In the following summer [1350], there was so great a lack of servants to do anything that, as one believed, there had hardly been so great a dearth in past times. For all the beasts and cattle that a man possessed wandered about without a shepherd, and everything a man had was without a caretaker. And so all necessities became so dear that anything that in the past had been worth a penny was now worth four or five pence. Moreover, both the magnates of the kingdom and the other lesser lords who had tenants, remitted something from the rents, lest the tenants should leave, because of the lack of servants and the dearth of things. Some remitted half the rent, some more and others less, some remitted it for two years, some for three, and others for one year, according as they were able to come to an agreement with their tenants. Similarly, those who received day-work from their tenants throughout the year, as is usual from serfs, had to release them and to remit such services. They either had to excuse them entirely or had to fix them in a laxer manner at a small rent, lest very great and irreparable damage be done to the buildings, and the land everywhere remain completely uncultivated. And all foodstuffs and all necessities became exceedingly dear.

Quoted in James B. Ross and Mary M. McLaughlin, eds., *The Portable Medieval Reader*. New York: Viking Press, 1949, pp. 216–22.

Document 6: A New Cemetery in London

Once the plague had entered England, in 1348, it quickly made its way to London. According to this tract from the chronicle of Robert of Avesbury, at the time a clerk employed in the Archbishop of Canterbury's court, the daily death toll became so large that authorities had to open a new burial ground.

The pestilence, which first began in the land inhabited by the Saracens [i.e., Muslims], grew so strong that, sparing no lordship, it visited every place in all the kingdoms stretching from that land northwards, up to and including Scotland, striking down the greater part of the people with the blows of sudden death. It began in England in the county of Dorset, about the feast of St Peter in chains [1 August], and immediately progressed without warning from place to place. It killed a great many healthy people, removing them from human concerns in the course of a morning. Those marked for death were scarcely permitted to live longer than three or four days. It showed favour to no one, except for a very few of the wealthy. On the same day 20, 40, or 60 bodies, and on many occasions many more, might be committed for burial together in the same pit.

The pestilence arrived in London at about the feast of All Saints [1 November] and daily deprived many of life. It grew so powerful that, between Candlemas [2 February, 1349] and Easter [12 April], more than 200 corpses were buried almost every day in the new burial ground made next to Smithfield, and this was in addition to the bodies buried in other churchyards in the city. It ceased in London with the coming of the grace of the Holy Spirit, that is to say at Pentecost [31 May], proceeding uninterrupted towards the north, where it also stopped about Michaelmas [29 September] 1349.

From *The Black Death*, by Rosemary Horrox (Manchester, UK: Manchester University Press, 1994). Reprinted by permission of the publisher.

Document 7: The Islamic World Engulfed by Plague

At the same time that the Black Death was devastating Italy, England, France, and other European lands, it was laying waste to neighboring Muslim regions in northern Africa and the Near East, as summarized here by the contemporary Muslim chronicler, Ibn Khaldun.

Civilization both in the East and the West was visited by a destructive plague which devastated nations and caused populations to vanish. It swallowed up many of the good things of civilization and wiped them out. It overtook the dynasties at the time of their senility, when they had reached the limit of their duration. It lessened their power and curtailed their influence. It weakened their authority. Their situation approached the point of annihilation and dissolution. Civilization decreased with the decrease of mankind. Cities and buildings were laid waste, roads and way signs were obliterated, settlements and mansions became empty, and dynasties and tribes grew weak. The entire inhabited world changed. The East, it seems, was similarly visited, though in accordance with and in proportion to [the East's more affluent] civilization. It was as if the voice of existence in the world had called out for oblivion and restriction and the world responded to its call. God inherits the earth and whoever is upon it.

Quoted in Robert S. Gottfried, *The Black Death: Natural and Human Disaster in Medieval Europe*. New York: Macmillan, 1983, pp. 41–42.

Popular Explanations for the Great Epidemic

Documents 8 and 9: The Pestilence Caused by Corrupted Air?

Besides the widely held theory that the Black Death was a divine punishment, alluded to in the writings of de Mussis and Boccaccio (see Documents 1 and 2), a number of physical causes were advanced to explain it. The following two fourteenth-century writings are among many that blame the great epidemic on corrupted, or foul, air emanating from a variety of sources. The first is by Florentine chronicler Matteo Villani, the other a section of the October 1348 report on the plague issued by the prestigious Paris Medical Faculty.

Having grown in vigor in Turkey and Greece and having spread thence over the whole Levant and Mesopotamia and Syria and Chaldea and Cyprus and Rhodes and all the islands of the Greek archipelago, the said pestilence leaped to Sicily, Sardinia and Corsica and Elba, and from there soon reached all the shores of the mainland. And of eight Genoese galleys which had gone to the Black Sea only four returned, full of infected sailors, who were smitten one after the other on the return journey. And all who arrived at Genoa died, and they corrupted the air to such an extent that whoever came near the bodies died shortly thereafter. And it was a disease in which there appeared certain swellings in the groin and under the armpit, and the victims spat blood, and in three days they were dead. And the priest who confessed the sick and those who nursed them so generally caught the infection that the victims were abandoned and deprived of confession, sacrament and medicine, and nursing. . . . And many lands and cities were made desolate.

Although major pestilential illnesses can be caused by the corruption of water or food, as happens at times of famine and infertility, yet we still regard illnesses proceeding from the corruption of the air as much more dangerous. This is because bad air is more noxious than food or drink in that it can penetrate quickly to the heart and lungs to do its damage. We believe that the present epidemic or plague has arisen from air corrupt in its substance, and not changed in its attributes. By which we wish it be understood that air, being pure and clear by nature, can only become putrid or corrupt by being mixed with something else, that is to say, with evil vapours. What happened was that the many vapours which had been corrupted at the time of the conjunction were drawn up from the earth and water, and were then mixed with the air and spread abroad by frequent gusts of wind in the wild southerly gales, and because of these alien vapours which they carried the winds corrupted the air in its substance, and are still doing so. And this corrupted air, when breathed in, necessarily penetrates to the heart and corrupts the substance of the spirit there and rots the surrounding moisture, and the heat thus caused destroys the life force, and this is the immediate cause of the present epidemic.

And moreover these winds, which have become so common here, have carried among us (and may perhaps continue to do so in future) bad, rotten and poisonous vapours from elsewhere: from swamps, lakes and chasms, for instance, and also (which is even more dangerous) from unburied or unburnt corpses—which might well have been a cause of the epidemic. Another possible cause of corruption, which needs to be borne in mind, is the escape of the rottenness trapped in the centre of the earth as a result of earthquakes—something which has indeed recently occurred. But the conjunctions could have been the universal and distant cause of all these harmful things, by which air and water have been corrupted.

Villani quoted in Robert S. Gottfried, *The Black Death: Natural and Human Disaster in Medieval Europe*. New York: Macmillan, 1983, p. 53; *Report of the Paris Medical Faculty, October 1348* from *The Black Death*, by Rosemary Horrox (Manchester, UK: Manchester University Press, 1994). Reprinted by permission of the publisher.

Document 10: Fumes Released by Earthquakes

A common medieval belief was that earthquakes released deadly fumes, a form of corrupted air, from beneath the earth and therefore that earthquakes were a direct cause of disease epidemics. This anonymous (probably German) document attributes the onset of the Black Death in 1348–1349 to earthquakes that had occurred in 1347.

It is a matter of scientific fact that earthquakes are caused by the exhalation of fumes enclosed in the bowels of the earth. When the fumes batter against the sides of the earth, and cannot get out, the earth is shaken and moves. I say that it is the vapour and corrupted air which has been vented—or so to speak purged—in the earthquake which occurred on St Paul's day, 1347, along with the corrupted air vented in other earthquakes and eruptions, which has infected the air above the earth and killed people in various parts of the world; and I can bring various reasons in support of this conclusion:

1. In Germany the mortality first began in Carinthia after an earthquake there in which the vapour and air enclosed deep in the mountains violently burst forth and hurled down mighty moun-

tains into the valleys, demolished the entire town of Villach, and buried numerous villages. And then the same mortality in turn invaded Austria, Hungary, Bavaria, Moravia, Bohemia, the Rhineland, Swabia and other provinces of Germany. Its progress followed no logical pattern; instead the filthy disease took a wandering and irregular route from place to place, as if blown along by the wind—something which can only be explained as the effect of corrupt air, expelled from the earth by the earthquake.

2. Houses near the sea, as at Venice and Marseilles, were affected quickly, as were low-lying towns on the edge of marshes or beside the sea, and the only explanation of that would seem to be the greater corruption of the air in hollows near the sea. . . .

4. It can be deduced from the corruption of fruit such as pears.

5. It can be deduced from the flooding of rivers, although this has been brought about by the heavy rain.

6. In every place where the mortality has persisted, virtually every victim has been afflicted as follows. For several days they spend most of each day asleep, weighed down by drowsiness, their heads made thick by a kind of fume, such as they might derive from eating or drinking fumous things. Most die within three days, although a few last for four. What happens is that when the poisonous fumes have gathered in the empty parts of the human body, especially in the chest, they rise into the head and trouble the animal spirits, which is one way of causing sleep.

7. In every place visited by the mortality the poor and common people die first, in great numbers, and the better off die later. But it is well known that the planets look down on rich and poor alike. The explanation would seem to be that the poor, who do not consume rich food or strong drink, do not generate heat or fumes inside themselves as the rich do, who are full of hot food and fumous drink. Therefore the rich do not so easily absorb fumes from outside, for what is inside them leaves no room for such fumes and blocks their entry.

From *The Black Death*, by Rosemary Horrox (Manchester, UK: Manchester University Press, 1994). Reprinted by permission of the publisher.

Document 11: Jews Poisoning Wells?

One contemporary theory for the onset of the Black Death, namely that Jews were involved in a massive conspiracy to poison Christian water supplies, led to tragedy. This excerpt from a document of that time chronicles just some of the hundreds of cruel and bloody anti-Semitic persecutions that swept Europe during the plague years.

The persecution of the Jews began in November 1348, and the first outbreak in Germany was at Sölden, where all the Jews were burnt on the strength of a rumour that they had poisoned wells and rivers, as was afterwards confirmed by their own confessions and also by the confessions of Christians whom they had corrupted and who had been induced by the Jews to carry out the deed. And some of the Jews who were newly baptised said the same. Some of these remained in the faith but some others relapsed, and when these were placed upon the wheel they confessed that they had themselves sprinkled poison or poisoned rivers. And thus no doubt remained of their deceitfulness which had now been revealed.

Within the revolution of one year, that is from All Saints [1 November] 1348 until Michaelmas [29 September] 1349 all the Jews between Cologne and Austria were burnt and killed for this crime, young men and maidens and the old along with the rest. And blessed be God who confounded the ungodly who were plotting the extinction of his church, not realising that it is founded on a sure rock and who, in trying to overturn it, crushed themselves to death and were damned for ever.

But now let us follow the killings individually. First Jews were killed or burnt in Sölden in November, then in Zofingen they were seized and some put on the wheel, then in Stuttgart they were all burnt. The same thing happened during November in Landsberg, a town in the diocese of Augsburg and in Bueron, Memmingen and Burgau in the same diocese. During December they were burnt and killed on the feast of St Nicholas [6 December] in Lindau, on 8 December in Reutlingen, on 13 December in Haigerloch, and on 20 December in Horw they were burnt in a pit. And when the wood and straw had been consumed, some Jews, both young and old, still remained half alive. The stronger of them snatched up cudgels and stones and dashed out the brains of those trying to creep out of the fire, and thus compelled those who wanted to escape the fire to descend to hell. And the curse seemed to be fulfilled: 'his blood be upon us and upon our children'.

On 27 December the Jews in Esslingen were burnt in their houses and in the synagogue. In *Nagelten* they were burnt. In the abovesaid town of Zofingen the city councillors, who were hunting for poison, found some in the house of a Jew called Trostli, and by experiment were satisfied that it was poison. As a result, two Jewish men and one woman were put on the wheel, but others were saved at the command of Duke Albrecht of Austria, who ordered that they should be protected. But this made little differ-

ence, for in the course of the next year those he had under his protection were killed, and as many again in the diocese of Constance.
But first those burnt in 1349 will be described in order.

Once started, the burning of the Jews went on increasing.
When people discovered that the stories of poisoning were un-
doubtedly true they rose as one against the Jews. First, on 2 January 1349 the citizens of Ravensburg burnt the Jews in the castle, to
which they had fled in search of protection from King Charles,
whose servants were imprisoned by the citizens after the burning.
On 4 January the people of Constance shut up the Jews in two of
their own houses, and then burnt 330 of them in the fields at sun-
set on 3 March. Some processed to the flames dancing, others
singing and the rest weeping. They were burnt shut up in a house
which had been specially built for the purpose. On 12 January in
Buchen and on 17 January in Basel they were all burnt apart from
their babies, who were taken from them by the citizens and baptised. They were burnt on 21 January in Messkirch and Waldkirch,
on 25 January in Speyer, and on 30 January in Ulm, on 11 February in Überlingen, on 14 February in the city of Strassburg (where
it took six days to burn them because of the numbers involved), on
16 February in Mengen, on 19th of the month in Sulgen, on 21st
in Schaffhausen and Zurich, on 23rd in St Gallen and on 3 March
in Constance, as described above, except for some who were kept
back to be burnt on the third day after the Nativity of the Virgin
[11 September].

Heinrich Truchess von Diessenhoven, *Persecution of the Jews*, from *The Black Death*, by Rosemary Horrox (Manchester, UK: Manchester University Press, 1994). Reprinted by permission
of the publisher.

Document 12: The Pope Defends the Jews

*Despite the widespread hysterical reactions to rumors blaming the plague
on the Jews, most religious and secular leaders realized that such rumors
were false, and some tried to stop the persecutions or protect Jews. This
order, issued on September 26, 1348, by Pope Clement VI, instructs all
members of the clergy to punish anyone taking part in anti-Jewish persecutions. Unfortunately, this and other similar orders were often ignored
by many Christians who, out of blind prejudice, ignorance, and terror,
committed unspeakable atrocities against thousands of innocent people.*

Although we rightly abhor the deceit of the Jews who, persisting
in their imperviousness [stubbornness], refuse to admit the secret
wisdom in the words of the prophets and their own writings or to
accept the Christian faith and salvation, we are nevertheless mind-

ful that Our Saviour chose to be born of Jewish stock when he put
on mortal flesh for the salvation of the human race, and that it is
our duty to succour humanity when the help of our protection and
the clemency of our Christian piety have been invoked. Accordingly, following in the footsteps of our predecessors of happy
memory, Popes Calixtus, Eugenius, Alexander, Clement, Celes-
tine, Innocent, Gregory, Nicholas, Honorius and Nicholas III, we
have taken the Jews under the shield of our protection, ordering
among the rest that no Christian presume in any wise to wound or
kill Jews, or take their money or expel them from his service before their term of employment has expired, unless by the legal
judgement of the lord or the officials of the country in which they
live; and that anyone who, knowing of these commands, still dares
to do the contrary, shall lose his title or office, or suffer the ultimate penalty of excommunication, unless he takes steps to correct
his presumption by making due satisfaction, as is set out more fully
in the letters.

Recently, however, it has been brought to our attention by public fame—or, more accurately, infamy—that numerous Christians
are blaming the plague with which God, provoked by their sins,
has afflicted the Christian people, on poisonings carried out by the
Jews at the instigation of the devil, and that out of their own hot-
headedness they have impiously slain many Jews, making no exception for age or sex; and that Jews have been falsely accused of
such outrageous behaviour so that they can be legitimately put on
trial before appropriate judges—which has done nothing to cool
the rage of the Christians but has rather inflamed them even more.
While such behaviour goes unopposed it looks as though their
error is approved.

Were the Jews, by any chance, to be guilty or cognizant of such
enormities a sufficient punishment could scarcely be conceived;
yet we should be prepared to accept the force of the argument that
it cannot be true that the Jews, by such a heinous crime, are the
cause or occasion of the plague, because throughout many parts of
the world the same plague, by the hidden judgement of God, has
afflicted and afflicts the Jews themselves and many other races who
have never lived alongside them.

We order you by apostolic writing that each of you upon whom
this charge has been laid, should straitly command those subject to
you, both clerical and lay, when they are assembled in worship at
mass, not to dare (on their own authority or out of hot-headedness)
to capture, strike, wound or kill any Jews or expel them from their

service on these grounds; and you should demand obedience under pain of excommunication, which henceforward you should use against those who disobey. But if they have ground of complaint against the Jews, whether concerning these matters or anything else, these letters in no way remove the power to proceed against them as was their right, but they should prosecute them in proper judicial form for these matters or any other offences before competent judges.

From *The Black Death*, by Rosemary Horrox (Manchester, UK: Manchester University Press, 1994). Reprinted by permission of the publisher.

Attempts to Deal with the Black Death

Document 13: An Herbal Treatment for the Plague

Since no one, including doctors, knew how to stop, prevent, or treat the plague, people tried a wide variety of approaches, both spiritual and physical, to combat it and prevent its spread. Of the numerous home remedies that sprang up, the following, often touted as a preventative measure, was one of the most popular.

A medicine for the pestilence. Take five cups of rue if it be a man, and if it be a woman leave out the rue, for rue is restorative to a man and wasting to a woman; and then take thereto five crops of tansey and five little blades of columbine, and a great quantity of marigold flowers full of the small chives from the crops that are like saffron chives. And if you may not get the flowers, take the leaves, and then you must have of the marigolds more than the others. Then take an egg that is newly laid, and make a hole in either end, and blow out all that is within. And lay it to the fire and let it roast till it may be ground to powder, but do not burn it. Then take a quantity of good treacle [substance used as a poison antidote], and bray all these herbs therein with good ale, but do not strain them. And then make the sick drink it for three evenings and three mornings. If they [the sick] hold it, they shall have life.

Quoted in Robert S. Gottfried, *The Black Death: Natural and Human Disaster in Medieval Europe.* New York: Macmillan, 1983, p. 116.

Document 14: Prayers to Save the Realm

As might be expected in a society as religiously devout as medieval Europe, when the Black Death struck prayer was widely seen as a potential means of fighting the disaster. At the time, prayers said by clergymen were perceived as having more weight with God than those said by everyday people.

So accordingly, for example, England's King Edward III asked John Stratford, the Archbishop of Canterbury, to order prayers by priests throughout the kingdom. When Stratford himself died of the pestilence, the duty fell on the Prior of Christchurch, who issued this document, usually referred to as Terribilis *(its opening word, Latin for "terrible").*

Terrible is God towards the sons of men, and by his command all things are subdued to the rule of his will. Those whom he loves he censures and chastises; that is, he punishes their shameful deeds in various ways during this mortal life so that they might not be condemned eternally. He often allows plagues, miserable famines, conflicts, wars and other forms of suffering to arise, and uses them to terrify and torment men and so drive out their sins. And thus, indeed, the realm of England, because of the growing pride and corruption of its subjects, and their numberless sins, has on many occasions stood desolate and afflicted by the burdens of the wars which are exhausting and devouring the wealth of the kingdom, and by many other miseries. And it is now to be feared that the same kingdom is to be oppressed by the pestilences and wretched mortalities of men which have flared up in other regions.

Our most excellent prince and lord, Edward by the grace of God the illustrious King of England and France, after giving serious consideration to these things, accordingly sent letters requesting John Stratford, formerly Archbishop of Canterbury, to have prayers said throughout the province of Canterbury for the peace of the church and of the realm of England, and so that Almighty God, of his ineffable mercy, might save and protect the king's realm of England from these plagues and mortality. But death stopped the archbishop putting the royal requests into practice. We, therefore, wishing, insofar as it pertains to us, to make good what he left unfinished, command and order you, on our authority as metropolitan of the church of Canterbury, to give strict instructions in all haste to every suffragan of our church of Canterbury that they, on our authority, urge and encourage those subject to them (or see that they are urged and encouraged) to intercede with the most high by devout prayers for these things. Bishops and others in priests' orders should celebrate masses and should organise, or have organised, sermons at suitable times and places, along with processions every Wednesday and Friday; and should perform other offices of pious propitiation humbly and devoutly, so that God, pacified by their prayers, might snatch the people of England from these tribulations, of his grace show help to them and, of his ineffable pity, preserve human frailty from these plagues and mortality.

And, so that those subject to you, and others within the province of Canterbury, should be made the more eager to do these things, you should arrange to grant indulgences to every one of your flock undertaking the things specified above. You should also, on our authority and that of our said church of Canterbury, tell all the other bishops to add indulgences on their own account, as seems best to them. You, meanwhile, are to see that all these things are effectively observed within your own city and diocese of London. Inform us in writing before Epiphany next when you received these letters and what action you took, and also tell your fellow-bishops to notify us in writing by the same date of the action they have taken.

From *The Black Death*, by Rosemary Horrox (Manchester, UK: Manchester University Press, 1994). Reprinted by permission of the publisher.

Document 15: A Mass to Drive Away the Plague

In addition to prayer, the Church tried holding special masses designed to ward off the pestilence. This popular one was called Salus populi.

Office: I am the safety of the people, says the Lord; when they shall have cried to me from tribulation I will hear them, and I shall be their Lord for ever.

Psalm 77: Attend, O my people, to my law: incline your ears to the words of my mouth.

Prayer: O God, who of your sole mercy removed the danger which hung over the people of Ninevah; to whom, so that you could show your mercy, you gave penitence and conversion; look, we beseech you, on your people prostrate before your mercy; for your mercy's sake, do not allow the people whom you redeemed with the blood of your only begotten son to die of pestilence [*mortalitatis*].

The Lesson (Jeremiah 14.7–8): If our iniquities have testified against us, O Lord, do thou it for thy name's sake, for our rebellions are many: we have sinned against thee. O expectation of Israel, the Saviour thereof in time of trouble. . . . But thou, O Lord, art among us, and thy name is called upon by us: forsake us not.

Gradual: Be kind, O Lord, to our sins; lest the people should say, 'Where is our God?'

Verse: Help us, O Lord our salvation; and for the honour of your name, O Lord, free us.

Alleluia: Lord, you are our refuge, from generation to generation.

The Gospel (Luke 11.9–13): At that time Jesus said to his disciples: Ask, and it shall be given you; seek, and you shall find; knock and it shall be opened to you. For everyone that asketh receiveth; and he that seeketh findeth; and to him that knocketh it shall be opened. And which of you, if he ask his father bread, will he give him a stone? Or a fish, will he for a fish give him a serpent? Or if he shall ask an egg, will he reach him a scorpion? If you then, being evil, know how to give good gifts to your children, how much more will your Father from heaven give the good Spirit to them that ask him?

Offertory: All who know your name, O Lord, trust in you; because you do not abandon those seeking you; sing unto the Lord who lives in Sion, for the cry of the poor is not forgotten.

Secret: Almighty God, look, we beseech you, favourably upon the gift of your church, and come before us in your mercy rather than your anger, for if you choose to take notice of our iniquities, no creature could survive it; but for the sake of the wonderful kindness with which you made us, do not let the works of your hand perish.

Communion: Amen I say to you: whatever you seek with prayers, believe that you will receive it; and be it done to you.

Post communion: Almighty and merciful God, look upon the people subject to your majesty; and may the receiving of your sacrament prevent the fury of cruel death from coming upon us.

From *The Black Death*, by Rosemary Horrox (Manchester, UK: Manchester University Press, 1994). Reprinted by permission of the publisher.

Document 16: Self-Punishment to Atone for Sin

Another spiritual approach to combating the Black Death was the one adopted by the flagellants—self-abuse. This excerpt from a contemporary chronicle, one of many that describe the flagellants, ends on a critical note, maintaining that the self-torturers erred by taking upon themselves the role of intermediary with God, and thereby challenged the Church's authority.

In 1348 a race without a head aroused universal wonder by their sudden appearance in huge numbers. They suddenly sprang up in all parts of Germany, calling themselves cross bearers or flagellants. They were said, as if in confirmation of the prophecy, to be without a head either because they literally had no head—that is to say no one to organise and lead them—or because they had no head in the sense of having no brain and no judgement; they were fools, laying claim to a form of piety but, as will appear, spoiling everything when their stupidities began to ferment. They were called cross bearers either because they followed a cross carried before them on their travels, or because they prostrated themselves in the form of a cross during their processions, or because they identified themselves with a cross stitched to their clothes. They were called flagellants because of the whips [*flagella*] which they used in performing public penance. Each whip consisted of a stick with three knotted thongs hanging from the end. Two pieces of needle-sharp metal were run through the centre of the knots from both sides, forming a cross, the ends of which extended beyond the knots for the length of a grain of wheat or less. Using these whips they beat and whipped their bare skin until their bodies were bruised and swollen and blood rained down, spattering the walls nearby. I have seen, when they whipped themselves, how sometimes those bits of metal penetrated the flesh so deeply that it took more than two attempts to pull them out.

Flocking together from every region, perhaps even from every city, they overran the whole land. In open country they straggled along behind the cross in no particular order, but when they came to cities, towns and villages they formed themselves into a procession, with hoods or hats pulled down over their foreheads, and sad and downcast eyes, they went through the streets singing a sweet hymn. In this fashion they entered the church and shut themselves in while they stripped off their clothes and left them with a guard. They covered themselves from the navel down with a pleated linen cloth like the women's undergarment which we call a kirtle, the upper part of the body remaining bare. Then they took the whips in their hands. When that was done, the north door of the church, if it had one, was opened. The eldest came out of the church first and threw himself to the ground immediately to the east of the door, beside the path. After him, the second lay down on the west side, then the third next to the first, the fourth next to the second and so on. Some lay with right hand raised, as though taking an oath, others lay on their belly or back, or on their right or left side, representing in this way the sins for which they were performing penance.

After this, one of them would strike the first with a whip, saying, 'May God grant you remission of all your sins. Arise'. And he would get up, and do the same to the second, and all the others in turn did the same. When they were all on their feet, and arranged two by two in procession, two of them in the middle of the column would begin singing a hymn in a high voice, with a sweet melody. They sang one verse and then the others took it up and repeated it after them, and then the singers sang the second verse and so on until the end. But whenever they came to the part of the hymn which mentioned the passion of Christ they all suddenly threw themselves down prostrate on the ground, regardless of where they were, and whether the ground was clean or filthy, whether there were thorns or thistles or nettles or stones. And they did not lower themselves gradually to their knees or steadying themselves in some other way, but dropped like logs, flat on their belly and face, with arms outstretched, and, lying there like crosses, would pray. A man would need a heart of stone to watch this without tears. At a sign given by one of them they would rise and resume their procession as before. And usually they sing the hymn three times, and prostrate themselves, as described, three times. And then, when they have returned to the same door by which they left the church, they re-enter and resume their clothes, taking off the linen cloths. As they leave the church they ask for nothing, re-questing neither food nor lodging, but accepting with gratitude the many offerings freely made to them.

However, just as annoying tares and persistent burrs often grow among the corn, so the ignorant and stupid, not content with penitential whippings, annoyingly and persistently took upon themselves the job of preaching. They did not think or speak of the clergy and the sacraments of the church with proper reverence, but rather with contempt; spat back rebukes and criticism, and despised persuasion. When they met up with two Dominicans in a field they were so infuriated by their exhortations that they tried to kill them, and although the more nimble managed to make his escape they stoned the other, and left his body under a pile of stones on the outskirts of Meissen. And they did similar things in many other places. . . .

The flagellants ignored and scorned the sentence of excommunication pronounced against them by bishops. They took no notice of the papal order against them—until princes, nobles and the more powerful citizens started to keep them at a distance. The people of Osnabrück never let them in, although their wives and other women clamoured for them. Afterwards they disappeared as suddenly as they had come, as apparitions or ghosts are routed by mockery.

From *The Black Death*, by Rosemary Horrox (Manchester, UK: Manchester University Press, 1994). Reprinted by permission of the publisher.

Document 17: Town Ordinances Attempt to Keep the Plague Out

A number of towns tried to limit the spread of the Black Death by imposing local regulations, including travel bans and various kinds of sanitary laws. The most complete surviving example comes from the northern Italian city of Pistoia, which issued its ordinances, some of which appear below, in May 1348. At the time, these were viewed as far-reaching and strict; however, because people were ignorant of the plague's actual modes of transmission, and did not eliminate or quarantine against infected rats and fleas, such regulations were largely ineffective. It is interesting to note that members of the upper classes were often exempt from certain restrictions, in the misguided belief that noble birth, title, wealth, and education would somehow protect against infection.

1. So that the sickness which is now threatening the region around Pistoia shall be prevented from taking hold of the citizens of Pistoia, no citizen or resident of Pistoia, wherever they are from or of what condition, status or standing they may be, shall dare or presume to go to Pisa or Lucca; and no one shall come to Pistoia from those places; penalty 500 pence. And no one from Pistoia shall receive or give hospitality to people who have come from those places; same penalty. And the guards who keep the gates of the city of Pistoia shall not permit anyone travelling to the city from Pisa or Lucca to enter; penalty 10 pence from each of the guards responsible for the gate through which such an entry has been made. But citizens of Pistoia now living within the city may go to Pisa and Lucca, and return again, if they first obtain permission from the common council—who will vote on the merits of the case presented to them. . . .

2. No one, whether from Pistoia or elsewhere, shall dare or presume to bring or fetch to Pistoia, whether in person or by an agent, any old linen or woollen cloths, for male or female clothing or for bedspreads; penalty 200 pence, and the cloth to be burnt in the public piazza of Pistoia by the official who discovered it. However it shall be lawful for citizens of Pistoia travelling within Pistoia and its territories to take linen and woollen cloths with them for their own use or wear, provided that they are in a pack or fardle weighing 30 lb or less. . . .

3. The bodies of the dead shall not be removed from the place of death until they have been enclosed in a wooden box, and the lid of planks nailed down so that no stench can escape, and covered with no more than one pall, coverlet or cloth; penalty 50 pence to

be paid by the heirs of the deceased or, if there are no heirs, by the nearest kinsmen in the male line. The goods of the deceased are to stand as surety for the payment of the penalty. Also the bodies are to be carried to burial in the same box; same penalty. . . .

4. To avoid the foul stench which comes from dead bodies each grave shall be dug two and a half armslength deep, as this is reckoned in Pistoia; penalty 10 pence from anyone digging or ordering the digging of a grave which infringes the statute.

5. No one, of whatever condition, status or standing, shall dare or presume to bring a corpse into the city, whether coffined or not; penalty 25 pence. And the guards at the gates shall not allow such bodies to be brought into the city; same penalty, to be paid by every guard responsible for the gate through which the body was brought.

6. Any person attending a funeral shall not accompany the corpse or its kinsmen further than the door of the church where the burial is to take place or go back to the house where the deceased lived, or to any other house on that occasion; penalty 10 pence. . . .

7. When someone dies, no one shall dare or presume to give or send any gift to the house of the deceased, or to any other place on that occasion, either before or after the funeral, or to visit the house, or eat there on that occasion; penalty 25 pence. This shall not apply to the sons and daughters of the deceased, his blood brothers and sisters and their children, or to his grandchildren. . . .

10. So that the sound of bells does not trouble or frighten the sick, the keepers of the campanile of the cathedral church of Pistoia shall not allow any of the bells to be rung during funerals, and no one else shall dare or presume to ring any of the bells on such occasions; penalty 10 pence, to be paid by the keepers who allowed the bells to be rung and by the heirs of the dead man, or his kinsmen should he have no heirs. When a parishioner is buried in his parish church or a member of a fraternity within the fraternity church the church bells may be rung, but only on one occasion and not excessively; same penalty. . . .

12. No one shall dare or presume to raise a lament or crying for anyone who has died outside Pistoia, or summon a gathering of people other than the kinsfolk and spouse of the deceased, or have bells rung, or use criers or any other means to invite people throughout the city to such a gathering; penalty 25 pence from each person involved.

However it is to be understood that none of this applies to the burial of knights, doctors of law, judges, and doctors of physic, whose bodies can be honoured by their heirs at their burial in any way they please. . . .

21. For the better preservation of health, there should be a ban on all kinds of poultry, calves, foodstuffs and on all kinds of fat being taken out of Pistoia by anybody; penalty 100 pence and the confiscation of the things being carried contrary to the ban. . . .

22. To avoid harm to men by stink and corruption, there shall in future be no tanning of skins within the city walls of Pistoia; penalty 25 pence. . . .

24. So that no corruption or stench should harm people's bodies, within the city the rendering down of dripping or suet should be done in houses at least 25 arms length from their neighbours and nowhere else; penalty 25 pence. . . .

33. Since wax for honouring the corpses of the dead cannot be found on sale, candles are not to be given, but instead it shall be permissible for anyone to give between 6 and 12 pence, at most, as he sees fit to each priest and friar who attends a funeral, in lieu of the candles and money which they were accustomed to give. But canons of the great church of Pistoia, prebendaries, priors, wardens and provosts of churches and of the orders of friars of Pistoia may be given twice that amount; penalty 25 pence.

34. The keepers of the fabric of each church in the city shall keep a supply of wax torches to be carried at the burial and to be held, alight, while the corpse is buried. And no other torches or wax lights should be held or carried at a burial; penalty 25 pence. And after the burial the torches shall be taken back and restored to the keepers, and they shall be reimbursed at the going rate for the wax used, with an additional 5 pence for the good of the dead person's soul.

From *The Black Death*, by Rosemary Horrox (Manchester, UK: Manchester University Press, 1994). Reprinted by permission of the publisher.

Chronology

1096–1099
Christian soldiers fight Muslims (or Saracens) in the Holy Land (Palestine) during the First Crusade, establishing major sea and land contacts between Europe and the East.

1223–1240
The Mongols (or Tartars), a central Asian people, invade and conquer what is now southern Russia.

1313
Giovanni Boccaccio, the Italian writer who will later pen the most famous description of the great plague, is born.

ca. 1320s
The Black Death, most likely bubonic plague, erupts somewhere in central Asia, probably in what is now Mongolia. The disease begins moving outward, following trade routes and other vectors of human habitation.

1345
The Black Death kills large numbers of Mongols in southern Russia.

1345–1346
The Mongols lay siege to Kaffa, a Genoese town on the Crimean Peninsula, along the northern shore of the Black Sea; the attackers hurl plague-infected bodies into the town; some of the Genoese escape and sail toward the Mediterranean, unaware that they are carrying the contagion with them.

1347
The Black Death arrives in Constantinople, Egypt, Sicily, and Italy.

1348
The pestilence reaches southern France, killing almost half the population of Avignon, temporary residence of the pope; many inland Italian cities, including Siena, Florence, Mantua, and Pistoia, feel the plague's wrath; over 200,000 people die as the plague ravages Egypt; the Black Death crosses the Alps into what is now Switzerland and Germany; it also moves northward through

France, killing hundreds of thousands in its path, and reaches the English Channel; the disease crosses the Channel and assaults England; the flagellant movement appears, probably in Germany, and spreads across the continent; Jews are accused of poisoning Christian wells and persecuted and murdered in large numbers.

1349
The Black Death reaches the Netherlands, Scotland, Ireland, and Scandinavia; Pope Clement VI calls for suppression of the flagellants.

1350
Slavic areas of Europe are devastated by the plague, which soon makes its way into northern Russia.

1351
The epidemic winds down, the disease apparently having run its course; the flagellants disperse in most areas, although a few bands survive for several more years.

1358
In the wake of rising labor costs and other economic difficulties brought on or worsened by the great epidemic, peasant uprisings occur in France.

1375
Boccaccio dies, leaving behind his *Decameron*, part of which describes the plague's onset in heart-rending detail; a secondary outbreak of plague occurs in England.

1664
An unexpected outbreak of the Black Death kills some 70,000 people in London.

1894
As still another outbreak of the bubonic plague runs its course in China, Swiss microbiologist Alexandre Yersin isolates the bacterium that causes the disease; he later develops a serum to treat it.

1900–1904
Bubonic plague appears in the U.S. city of San Francisco; 121 people are infected and all but three die.

1994
Over fifty people die when the plague reappears in India.

For Further Research

Primary Sources on the Black Death

Editor's Note: The only major, substantial collection of original documents pertaining to the Black Death presently available is Rosemary Horrox, ed., *The Black Death*. Manchester, Eng.: Manchester University Press, 1994. A few dozen lengthy primary source quotes appear in Robert S. Gottfried's *The Black Death* (see below), while most standard collections of medieval documents, such as *The Portable Medieval Reader* (James B. Ross and Mary M. McLaughlin, eds., New York: Viking Press, 1949) and *Readings in European History* (Leon Bernard and Theodore B. Hodges, eds., New York: Macmillan, 1958), contain only one or two each. Among the single contemporary accounts of the Black Death, two of the longest and most detailed are those by Giovanni Boccaccio in his *Decameron* and the French chronicler Jean de Venette. Important late medieval works that describe post-plague society and attitudes include Geoffrey Chaucer's famous *Canterbury Tales*; William Langland's *Piers the Ploughman*; and John Froissart's *Chronicles of England, France, and Spain*.

European Society on the Eve of the Black Death

Bruce M.S. Campbell, ed., *Before the Black Death: Studies in the "Crisis" of the Early Fourteenth Century*. Manchester, England: University of Manchester Press, 1991.

George Holmes, *The Later Middle Ages, 1272–1485*. New York: W.W. Norton, 1962. Note: This volume also contains a short section on the effects of the Black Death on medieval peasants.

Marjorie Rowling, *Life in Medieval Times*. New York: Berkley Publishing, 1968. Note: This volume also contains a short section describing the onset of the Black Death.

R.W. Southern, *The Making of the Middle Ages*. New Haven, CT: Yale University Press, 1953.

Barbara W. Tuchman, *A Distant Mirror: The Calamitous 14th Century*. New York: Knopf, 1978.

General Studies of the Fourteenth-Century Onset of the Black Death

William M. Bowsky, *The Black Death: A Turning Point in History?* New York: Holt, Rhinehart and Winston, 1971.

Ann G. Carmichael, *Plague and Poor in Renaissance Florence.* Cambridge: Cambridge University Press, 1986.

Phyllis Corzine, *The Black Death.* San Diego: Lucent Books, 1997.

Michael W. Dols, *The Black Death in the Middle East.* Princeton, NJ: Princeton University Press, 1977.

Robert S. Gottfried, *The Black Death: Natural and Human Disaster in Medieval Europe.* New York: Macmillan, 1983.

David Herlihy, *The Black Death and the Transformation of the West.* Ed. Samuel K. Cohn Jr. Cambridge, MA: Harvard University Press, 1997.

Geoffrey Marks, *The Medieval Plague: The Black Death of the Middle Ages.* Garden City, NY: Doubleday, 1971.

Johannes Nohl, *The Black Death: A Chronicle of the Plague.* Trans. C.H. Clarke. New York: Harper and Row, 1969.

Colin Platt, *King Death: The Black Death and Its Aftermath in Late-Medieval England.* Toronto: University of Toronto Press, 1997.

J.F.D. Shrewsbury, *A History of the Bubonic Plague in the British Isles.* Cambridge: Cambridge University Press, 1970.

Philip Ziegler, *The Black Death.* New York: Harper and Row, 1969.

Social, Economic, and Psychological Effects of the Black Death and Other Disease Epidemics

Jon Arrizabalaga et al., eds., *The Great Pox: The French Disease in Renaissance Europe.* New Haven, CT: Yale University Press, 1997.

Maurice Beresford and John G. Hurst, eds., *Deserted Medieval Villages.* New York: St. Martin's Press, 1971.

Samuel J. Cohn Jr., *The Cult of Remembrance and the Black Death: Six Renaissance Cities in Central Italy.* Baltimore: Johns Hopkins University Press, 1992.

Otto Freidrich, *The End of the World: A History.* New York: Fromm International, 1986.

John Hatcher, *Plague, Population and the English Economy, 1348–*

1530. London: Macmillan, 1977.

George Huppert, *After the Black Death: A Social History of Early Modern Europe*. Bloomington: Indiana University Press, 1986.

Maurice Keen, *English Society in the Later Middle Ages, 1348–1500*. New York: Penguin Books, 1990.

Mark Ormrod and Philip Lindley, eds., *The Black Death in England*. Stamford: Paul Watkins, 1996.

Terence Ranger and Paul Slack, eds., *Epidemics and Ideas: Essays on the Historical Perception of Pestilence*. Cambridge: Cambridge University Press, 1992.

Jeffrey Richards, *Sex, Dissidence and Damnation: Minority Groups in the Middle Ages*. New York: Barnes and Noble, 1990.

John Walter and Roger Schofield, eds., *Famine, Disease and Social Order in Early Modern Society*. Cambridge: Cambridge University Press, 1989.

Physical Causes, Effects, and Treatments of Plague and Other Diseases

Frederick F. Cartwright and Michael D. Biddiss, *Disease and History*. New York: Dorset Press, 1972.

James C. Giblin, *When Plague Strikes: The Black Death, Smallpox, AIDS*. New York: HarperCollins, 1995.

Charles T. Gregg, *Plague: An Ancient Disease in the Twentieth Century*. Albuquerque: University of New Mexico Press, 1985.

Howard W. Haggard, *The Doctor in History*. New York: Dorset Press, 1989.

Arno Karlen, *Man and Microbes: Disease and Plagues in History and Modern Times*. New York: G.P. Putnam's Sons, 1995.

William H. McNeill, *Plagues and Peoples*. New York: Doubleday, 1977.

Katherine Park, *Doctors and Medicine in Early Renaissance Florence*. Princeton, NJ: Princeton University Press, 1985.

Henry Sigerist, *Civilization and Disease*. New York: Cornell University Press, 1943.

Graham Twigg, *The Black Death: A Biological Reappraisal*. New York: Schocken Books, 1984.

Hans Zinsser, *Rats, Lice and History*. Boston: Little, Brown, 1935.

Index

AIDS, 116, 119, 124, 125
Albert II (duke of Austria), 89
animals
  attacks on corpses by, 52
  disease transmitted by, 31–32, 122, 125
  plague transmitted by, 35–36
anti-Semitism. *See* Jews
architecture, 104, 107–108
Arles, 55
Asia, 15
  plague in, 42–44, 45
  travel to, 39
astrology, 57–58, 60
Athenian Plague, 33
Avignon, 46, 55

babesiosis, 120
Bacon, Roger, 113
Bartolus of Sassoferrato, 82
Berlin, 54
Biddiss, Michael D., 109
Black Death
  as bubonic plague, 13, 14–15
  causes of
    Jews as, 19–21, 82–84
    saints as, 81–82
    and superstitions, 57–58
    theories on, 17–19
  as contagious, 62–63, 71
  control of, 65–66, 70–72
    ordinances for, 66–68
    quarantines for, 68–70
  deaths from, 11, 21, 48, 54–55
    graphic expression of, 53–54
    and rich vs. poor, 100
  effects of, 11–12, 21–23
    architectural, 104, 107–108
    demographic, 94–95, 98–101
    economic, 92–94, 95–96
    and land redistribution, 106–107
    on languages, 103–105, 110–12
    on religion, 24–25
    technological, 23–24, 97–98
    on universities, 105–106
  Europe on eve of, 38–39, 91–92
  flight from, 63–64

  origin of, 41–42
  suffering from, reports on, 49–53
  survivors of, 53
  transmission of, 13–14, 15–17, 42–47
  see also plague
Boccaccio, Giovanni, 11, 12, 46, 49
  on burials, 52
  on flight from Black Death, 92–93
  on God's wrath, 18
Bordeaux, 46
Bristol, 55–56
Brotherhood of Flagellants, 74
bubonic plague. *See* plague, bubonic
Burgundy, 46
burials, 66, 67
  lack of, 52–53
  and sanitation laws, 67–68
  see also gravediggers

Cambridge University, 105–106
Carmichael, Ann G., 65
Cartwright, Frederick F., 109
Catholic Church
  effect of Black Death on, 24–25, 110–12
  and flagellants, 20–21, 78
  influence of, 109–10
  and Jews, 83, 84, 86
  and medicine, 60–62, 112–13
Centers for Disease Control, 122
Charles IV (emperor), 79
Chauliac, Guy de, 55, 60, 64
children
  demographics of, 94–95
  orphaned, 50–52
China. *See* Asia
chlamydia, 119
cholera, 31
Christians. *See* Catholic Church
Clement VI (pope), 21, 87
  and flagellants, 79–80
Constantinople, 16
Covino, Simon de, 62–63
Cremona, 54
Crusades, 83
Cyprus, 56

170

Defoe, Daniel, 49
demographics, 94–95, 98–100
dengue shock syndrome, 124
diarrhea, 31
diphtheria, 31, 119
diseases
  during classical/medieval times,
    33–35
  immunity to, 32–33
  new, 115–17, 118–23
  sexually transmitted, 123–24
  source of, 124–26
  transmission of, 30–32
  see also Black Death; plague
Dols, Michael W., 41
dysentery, 31

Ebola, 121–22
encephalitis viruses, 121
England, 46
  deaths in, 55–56
  languages in, 104–105
epidemics. See diseases; plague
epizootics, 14, 32
Europe
  before Black Death, 29–30
  on eve of Black Death, 38–39,
    91–92
  transmission of Black Death to,
    15–17, 44–47

Fayt, Jean da, 79
fires, 59, 62
flagellants, 20–21, 74–75
  and the Church, 78–80
  precedence to, 73–74
  suffering by, 75–78
fleas, 13, 15, 36, 37–38
Florence, 46
  deaths in, 55–56
  demographics in, 94–95
Foligno, Gentile da, 60, 63
France, 54, 55
Friedrich, Otto, 73

Galen (physician), 34, 71, 113
Genoa, 15, 43, 46
  deaths in, 56
Germany, 46
  deaths in, 49, 54–55
God
  faith in, 25
  punishment by, 12

wrath of, 17–18, 81–82
  see also flagellants
Golden Horde, 45
Gonzaga, Ludovico, 69
Gottfried, Robert S., 22, 29
Gower, John, 22–23
gravediggers
  demand for, 93
  Jews as, 86
Guillain-Barré syndrome, 122
Gutenberg, Johann, 98

Harvey, William, 113
hemorrhagic fever, 120, 121–22, 124
Henry II (king of England), 111
Henson, Jim, 123
Herlihy, David, 14, 17, 91
herpes, 119, 123–24
Hippocrates, 59
Hoitfeld, Arrid, 53
Horrox, Rosemary, 13, 15
human papilloma virus (HPV), 124
Hungary, 47
Huss, John, 111

Ibn al-Wardi, 42, 44
Iceland, 56
India, 15, 44, 116
influenza, 31, 117
Innocent III (pope), 84, 86
Ireland, 46
Italy
  deaths in, 55–56
  plague control in, 71

Janibeg (Kipchak khan), 45
Jesus Christ, 76
Jews
  efforts to protect, 87–88
  human rights of, 84
  massacres of, 88–89
  as moneylenders, 84–85
  persecution of, 19–20, 82–84
  restrictions against, 85–87
Joachim of Fiore, 74
Junin virus, 120

Kaffa, 44, 45
Karlen, Arno, 115
Knighton, Henry, 23

labor, 93, 97
Langland, William, 110

languages, 103–104
Lassa fever, 121
Legionnaires' disease, 122–23
leprosy, 39, 82–83
Lollards, the, 111
London, 55–56
Lorraine, 54
Luther, Martin, 111
Lyme disease, 119, 121
Lyons, 46

malaria, 30, 39
  reappearance of, 118
Malthus, Thomas, 99
Marburg disease, 120
Marks, Geoffrey, 57
Marseilles, 46, 55
  deaths in, 50
Massis, Gilles de, 55
measles, 31, 34–35, 39
  reappearance of, 118, 119
medicine, 24
  influence of Church on, 60–62,
    112–13
  optimism in, 117–18
  and superstition, 57–60
  theory on contagion, 62–63
Merton College, 106
Messina, 43, 45
Michael of Piazza, 43, 45
Middle Ages
  diseases during, 31
    immunity to, 32–33
    origin of, 33–35
  living conditions of, 29–30
  population during, 99–100
  social classes during, 100–101
Middle East, 42, 44
Milan, 54, 70, 71
Mongols, 15–16, 45
Moscow, 54
Mussi, Gabriele de', 44–45

Naples, 54–55
nationalism, 104–105
New College, 106
Nohl, Johannes, 48
Novgorod, 54

Oxford University, 103, 106

pandemic, 38
Paris, 46

College of Physicians, 57
peasants, 22–23
Perugia, 67
pestilence, 117
Pevsner, Nikolaus, 104
Philip (king of France), 79
Philippe de Valois (king of France),
  57
physicians
  on cause of plague, 57–58
  demand for, 93
  flight of, 64
Pisa, 46
Pistoia, 18–19, 66
plague, 39
  bubonic, 32, 36–37
    Black Death as, 13, 14–15
    reappearance of, 118
  as contagious, 71
  environmental conditions for,
    37–38
  pneumonic, 30, 31, 37
  septicaemic, 37
  transmission of, 35–36
  see also Black Death; diseases
pogroms, 89
  see also Jews
Poland, 47
polyptych, 100
priests
  demand for, 93
  loss of, 110
  in universities, 105–106
printing, 23–24, 98
Protestant Reformation, 111–12

quarantines, 18–19, 68–70, 72

Ragusa, 68
Raniero (hermit), 73
rats. See rodents
Renaissance, 113
Richard II (king of England), 23
Righi, Alessandro, 100–101
Robert of Avesbury, 77
Roch, Saint, 81, 112
rodents, 13, 15, 35–36, 41–42
  see also animals
Roman Empire, 34
Rome, 54
Rupert of the Palatinate, 89
Russia, 15
rype, the, 53

sanitary conditions, 31
    legislation on, 65, 66, 67–68
Scotland, 46
sea trade, 33–34, 39
    transmission of Black Death
        through, 42–44, 45–46
shipping, 24
Sicily, 46
Simon Sudbury (archbishop of
    Canterbury), 111
smallpox, 34, 39
Stewart, William H., 118
surgery, 61–62
swine flu virus, 122
syphilis, 118, 119

technology, 23–24, 97–98
Thomas Aquinas, Saint, 84
Thurgau, 54
Toulon, 55
toxic-shock-like syndrome (TSLS),
    123
toxic shock syndrome, 123
travel
    bans on, 67, 70, 71–72
    and quarantining, 68–69
    and sea trade, 33–34
tuberculosis, 119
Tuchman, Barbara, 20–21, 81

Turin, 54
Tuscany, 67
    demographics in, 94, 95
Twigg, Graham, 14
typhoid, 31
typhus, 117

universities
    establishment of, 105–106
    loss of, 103

Venette, Jean de, 16
Venice, 19, 46, 54
    deaths in, 55–56
Vienna, 55
Villani, Matteo, 95, 100
viruses, 119, 121
Visconti, Bernabò, 69, 70
Visconti, Filippo Maria, 71
Visconti, Giangaleazzo, 70
Visconti, Gian Maria, 71

whooping cough, 119
William of Wykeham, 106
women, 93–94
Wyclif, John, 110

Ziegler, Philip, 46, 102